Treading in the Past

/// \\\ /// \\\ /// \\\ /// \\\ /// \\\ /// \\\ /// \\\ /// \\\ /// \\\ /// \\\ /// \\\ /// \\\ ///

Treading in the Past

Sandals of the Anasazi

/// \\\ /// \\\ /// \\\ /// \\\ /// \\\ /// \\\ /// \\\ /// \\\ /// \\\ /// \\\ /// \\\ /// \\\ /// \\

EDITED BY **Kathy Kankainen**

PHOTOGRAPHS BY **Laurel Casjens**

A Catalog of the
Anasazi Sandal
Collection at the
Utah Museum of
Natural History

/// \\\ /// \\\ /// \\\

*Supported by
grants from the
Herbert I. and
Elsa B. Michael
Foundation,
Frances Holliday
Minton, and Teva
Sport Sandals*

Utah Museum of Natural History
in association with the
University of Utah Press
Salt Lake City

Copublished by the Utah Museum of Natural History and the University of Utah Press.

Printed in Korea

LIBRARY OF CONGRESS CATALOGING-IN-PUBLICATION DATA

Utah Museum of Natural History.
   Treading in the past : sandals of the Anasazi / edited by Kathy Kankainen ; photography by Laurel Casjens.
      p.   cm.
   "A catalog of the Anasazi Sandal Collection at the Utah Museum of Natural History."
   "Utah Museum of Natural History in Association with the University of Utah Press.
   Includes bibliographical references.
   ISBN 0–87480–470–1 (cloth). — ISBN 0–87480–471–X (pbk.)
   1. Pueblo Indians—Costume—Catalogs.   2. Sandals—Southwest, New—Catalogs.   3. Pueblo Indians—Antiquities—Catalogs.   4. Utah Museum of Natural History—Catalogs.   I. Kankainen, Kathy, 1944–   II. Casjens, Laurel.   III. Title.
E99.P9U83 1995
391'.413—dc20   94-25169

CONTENTS

/// \\\ //

FOREWORD

Various species of yucca plants are found throughout the Southwest. They are tough, persistent, slow growing. Their roots are stout. They flourish in landscapes familiar to any westerner: sandy sites in warm desert shrub, sagebrush, pinyon-juniper, and ponderosa pine communities. Their flowers can be spectacular; botanists call them "large and showy, numerous, perfect." They are the fiber source, the mother plants for virtually all the sandals in this book.

It is irresistible to liken this publication to a yucca plant. Here is the inflorescence of years of quiet work and persistent growth of the study and documentation of prehistoric textiles at the Utah Museum of Natural History.

The museum's Textile Laboratory has been staffed primarily by museum-trained volunteers. Many are fiber artists recruited from the membership of the Mary M. Atwater Weavers Guild. Because they make textiles themselves, they bring a kind of organic understanding about the ways fibers are twisted and spun and interlaced to create sandals, baskets, and cloth. They bring perseverance (three celebrated their fifteenth year at the museum in 1995) and a capacity to thrive in seemingly low nutrient terrain (the laboratory began in a converted men's room in the old Stewart School at the University of Utah) and to create something beautiful and enduring. They are responsible for this project.

It gives me great pleasure to name them: Kristina F. Burton, Kathy Kankainen, Sue Ellen Lee, Becky Menlove, Frances H. Minton, Vilah Jean Peterson, and Jane Tomb.

It also pleases me to acknowledge the generous, nourishing, and enduring support of the Steiner Foundation. The foundation's board has made an annual contribution to the Textile Laboratory since 1981. They, too, are responsible for the success of the laboratory.

Under a polarizing light microscope, yucca is beautiful: it is brilliant and crystalline and moves light the way an icicle does. One thinks of Spider Woman, who taught the Navajo people to weave on a loom of sun rays and halos, of rock crystal and lightning and rain streamers. And then one thinks of the Anasazi weavers, the ones who made these exquisite sandals. Their silent presence inhabits this book.

We cannot name them, but we honor them.

Ann Hanniball

ACKNOWLEDGMENTS

The staff of the Textile Laboratory at the Utah Museum of Natural History, past and present, are truly exceptional and dedicated people. Working with them has been an honor—as working with the sandals has been. We have all felt the enduring human relationships they represent and have spent quiet moments just sharing space with a sandal.

Ann Hanniball, past curator of collections and now assistant director of the museum, was the energizing force behind this project. Her expertise, persistence, and deep belief in the importance of textiles in prehistory have made this publication a reality. Sharing her passion for textiles and their inquiry are Textile Laboratory volunteers Jane M. Tomb, Vilah Jean Peterson, Frances H. Minton, Sue Ellen Lee, and Kristina F. Burton. Past supervisor Becky Menlove was instrumental in organizing and laying out initial plans for the book as well as creating the title. Laurel Casjens, present curator of collections and photographer for the book, not only lent her photographic skills but served as a constant support. Tina Roe's computer expertise was vital in producing this manuscript.

We are indebted to the staff of the University of Utah Press, especially Jeff Grathwohl, for their enthusiasm and assistance in this project. Drew Ross, manager of the Marriott Library archives, was most helpful in obtaining historic photographs. In addition, support from the Utah Museum of Natural History, its staff, and its director, Sarah George, is greatly appreciated. This project would not have been possible without the financial support of the Herbert I. and Elsa B. Michael Foundation, Frances Holliday Minton and Teva Sport Sandals, for which we are deeply grateful. I personally value the support of my friends and family, especially Eric.

The real kudos go to the Anasazi who produced this rich material culture. They have left a legacy of textile weaving for us to ponder, ravel, spin, and reweave.

Kathy Kankainen

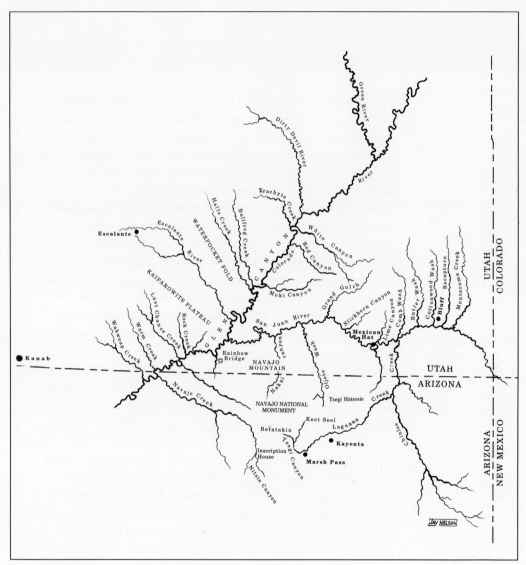

Four Corners area

Introduction

This book takes readers on a journey into a prehistoric culture in which people's daily activities hinged on their ability to utilize the environment for survival and aesthetic success.

From approximately A.D. 1 to 1300, the people we now refer to as *Anasazi* inhabited parts of Utah, Colorado, Arizona, and New Mexico. They left pecked and painted images on rock surfaces and an extraordinary number of artifacts and architectural ruins that reveal their genius in building, farming, and ceramics. The Anasazi were also skilled textile artists, producing loomed clothes, intricate baskets, and sandals. We are fortunate that so many of their perishable artifacts survived because of the arid climate of the Four Corners region.

The term *weaving* applies to techniques that interlace two or more fibers or sets of fiber elements. Sandal makers used other methods as well, but applied them in conjunction with weaving. Working with fibers, whether to produce cloth, baskets, or sandals, was closely intertwined with Anasazi survival. It seems appropriate to call the Anasazi weavers textile artists.

Two types of a desert plant called yucca—narrow-leaf and broad-leaf—were the most common sources of fiber for Anasazi artisans. The leaves of the yucca plant were used whole, split, or separated, or they could be shredded and then spun and twisted into cordage. Cordage became both warp (vertical threads) and weft (horizontal threads) for fine, intricately designed sandals. Sandal makers added ties and loops of leaves and cordage to secure the sandals to the wearer's feet.

The earliest Anasazi sandals excavated by archaeologists are from the Basketmaker II period (A.D. 1–500). These sandals have square heels and toes woven in a complex twining and wrapping technique.

The most intricate and finely woven sandals come from the Basketmaker III period (A.D. 500–700). Their toes are scalloped and their heels puckered. These cordage sandals exhibit a complex weave with a smooth, ribbed surface on the interior and a raised geometric pattern on the sole. Such a tread pattern would have been practical for crossing hot, difficult terrain or scaling cliff walls. But if practicality were the only consideration, such exquisite designs would have been unnecessary. Perhaps these designs sprang from a maker's pure pleasure in the ability to create something beautiful. Some weavers from the Basketmaker III period used natural dyes and mineral pigments to color their weft cordage and produced elegant, multicolored geometric designs.

Weavers of the Pueblo I (A.D. 700–900) and Pueblo II (A.D. 900–1100) periods produced coarse cordage sandals with rounded or pointed toes. Sandals dated to the Pueblo II and Pueblo III (A.D. 1100–1300) periods were plaited of yucca leaves, some with toe jogs. Other types in abundance during Pueblo II and Pueblo III times were plain weave sandals woven with whole, split, or separated leaf elements for warp and weft.

Since the early 1900s the University of Utah and other institutions have sponsored archaeological expeditions in the Southwest. Archaeologists have discovered, surveyed, excavated, and documented prehistoric sites, collecting artifacts for further research. Their fieldwork has produced hundreds of thousands of specimens, site notes, and related material, some of it now deposited in the Utah Museum of Natural History. Among the artifacts are the 308 Anasazi sandals and sandal fragments that are the focus of this book.

The majority of the sandals in the museum's anthropological collection were gathered in the early 1900s by Byron Cummings, a pioneering southwestern archaeologist. Another eighty-one of them were collected during the Upper Colorado River Basin Archaeological Salvage Project (UCRBASP) in the 1950s, under the direction of Jesse Jennings. This project, also called the Glen Canyon project, was one of "emergency archaeology." Its goal was to extract as much information as possible from Glen Canyon sites before the Colorado River was dammed to form Lake Powell. The remaining sandals in the collection came from a variety of other expeditions to southern Utah.

Not surprisingly, most of the sandals presented in this book show some type of wear. Worn or missing heels are most common. On others, slight indentations on the interior mark where someone's foot or toe rested. Yet even a small fragment may have a start, finish, tie, or knot that can tell a story. Small details help the observer reconstruct what Anasazi hands wove years ago. This connection of past to present gives life to every sandal.

Dating sandals, especially those collected during the Cummings era, is difficult. Most sandals in this collection are dated by the presence (or absence) of benchmark pottery types found at the same site or portion of a site as the sandals. Thus they can be dated only if their location was accurately recorded. Radiocarbon dating is possible but destructive, because a large sample must be taken from each sandal for testing.

The following four essays on textiles, archaeology, plant materials, and methods of manufacture explore the Anasazi and their sandal weaving techniques and offer a glimpse of the two archaeologists who contributed most to this collection. In the catalog that follows, specimens are organized by site of origin. In the stunning photographs by Laurel Casjens, the sandals are all pictured with toe toward the top of the page.

This book presents the sandals and accompanying documentation to provide insight into the Anasazi and to encourage further study. The impact of the sandals as a group is emotionally and aesthetically powerful—a tribute to Anasazi sandal weavers.

Kathy Kankainen

Anasazi Textiles

Elizabeth A. Morris   /// \\\ /// \\\ /// \\\ /// \\\ /// \\\ /// \\\ /// \\\ /// \\\ /// \\\ /// \\\ /// \\\ ///

The modern traveler passing through the rugged uplands and colorful canyons of the southwestern United States may not be aware that this desert country has preserved rare evidence of usually perishable prehistoric artifacts. Leather, wood, foodstuffs, feathers, and fiber fashioned into containers, farming implements, weapons, bedding, and clothing reflect skilled use of locally harvested materials. The makers—the Anasazi—made their homes in sandy flats and shallow rock shelters in the towering cliffs. Modern Pueblo tribes of Arizona and New Mexico are among their descendants. Protected from the deteriorating effects of weather and climate, a large variety of cultural materials has survived to provide irreplaceable insight into the lifeways of the Anasazi.

Utah, Arizona, New Mexico, and Colorado offer one of the richest reflections of the lifestyles of ancient peoples available anywhere in the world. The conditions of preservation and the sophistication of technologies such as fine sandal weaving compare favorably with those of famous objects from Mexico, Peru, and Egypt. Dating from throughout the last two thousand years, some of the finest examples of sandals were made between the fourth and the thirteenth centuries A.D. The desert environment, the respect and reverence of its native inhabitants, and the relatively sparse modern population helped preserve these remains until they came to the attention of scientists early in the twentieth century.

Perhaps best known among the creative efforts of the Anasazi are the numerous rock art panels and impressive architectural remains in open sites and shallow caves. These have received more attention and study and, indeed, are easier to find and appreciate than are artifacts such as sandals in museum collections. This volume is the most comprehensive text on sandals published to date. Communicating the complex fiber manipulations involved in weaving is indispensable to understanding the Anasazi. Weaving was extensively practiced and vital to survival.

In addition to yucca fibers, many other materials were utilized by these ancient people. Artifacts of human, dog, and wild animal hair, bast fibers such as milkweed, apocynum, mesquite, and cliff rose, and the bark of willow and juniper are all part of the archaeological inventory. Cotton occurs rarely in early Anasazi contexts and more commonly in later times. A useful technique for making warm blankets and robes consisted of twisting narrow, supple elements of split feathers and furry hides around the structural elements of coarse, netlike fabrics woven of yucca string. Sometimes brightly colored songbird feathers were used decoratively on the edges and corners of the blankets.

Besides blankets and sandals, the list of garments includes leggings, socks, belts, aprons, kilts, and, rarely, shirts. Other archaeological objects include mats, baskets, tump bands, quivers, game nets, and bags. Some of these were made of coarse, hardly altered raw materials such as yucca leaves and juniper bark, while others were finely woven of carefully prepared string.

Nonloomed fabrics are most common in collections of Anasazi objects. After A.D. 1000, evidence of looms and associated weaving tools is found. Plain weaving, plaiting, twining, netting, openwork, and tapestry techniques were among the wide variety of weaving technologies.

Textiles were sometimes decorated beyond the manufacturing process. Mineral and vegetal colors—red, yellow, black, white, and, more rarely, blue and green—were used to dye woven elements or occasionally to create painted or tie-dyed designs. Embroidery was also used as decoration.

Sandals are one category of fiber artifact that occurs in particular abundance. They were found in ruins that mostly date between A.D. 400 and 1300. Because the earlier Anasazi made beautiful baskets and did not make pottery, they were named Basketmakers. Together with leather moccasins and socks made of human hair in a looping technique, there have been found hundreds of items of footgear made from parts of yucca plants. Some are plaited or plain weave using whole or split leaves. Many are constructed of carefully prepared yucca fiber yarn.

Not only were sandals made in different techniques, many also incorporated colorful geometric patterns and reveal elaborate manipulations of warp and weft elements to provide a raised sole pattern. Within the relatively rigid requirements of size, shape, and function, sandal makers created almost as many decorative expressions as there are recorded specimens. Although there are similarities in the details of manufacture and decoration of these fine types, no two identical specimens have been discovered so far. Each one is unique.

Yucca plants and the fibers derived from their sharp leaves may seem unlikely raw materials for articles of clothing. This shrub, which includes species of the genus *Yucca*, grows abundantly in the dry, sandy soil of the American Southwest. Its spiked leaves and woody composition resist attacks by all except

Yucca in bloom (photo
by Laurel Casjens)

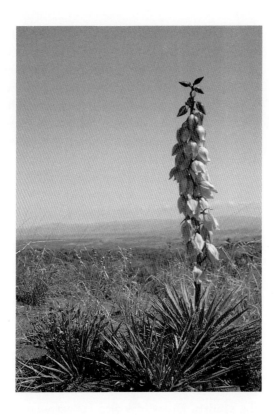

the cleverest of animals who browse the plant parts when
absolutely necessary. Only the creamy white flowers are easily
harvested by the casual collector.

When the leaves are used as cut from the stem, they are
numerous, straight, and strong. Additionally, the abrasive, hard-
surfaced leaves contain a sheaf of long, contiguous fibers running
separately from end to end. When cut, soaked, and scraped by
the Basketmaker people they yielded excellent hanks of fiber
suitable for spinning into strong yarn, strings, or rope of a wide
variety of diameters. When the clean fiber was further soaked
and pounded until it split, it could be even finer, softer, and
more supple to manipulate. Fibers were then spun into single
yarns that were often further twisted together to form two-
and three-ply yarn. The end products of the finest of processing
compare favorably with the natural and synthetic fibers utilized
in our clothing today. The sophistication of many of these
remnants of prehistoric textile manufacture attests to the high
quality of the techniques used and to the cultural standards of
excellence.

Not only was dyed yarn woven into complex, geometric,
colored designs, there also were intricate weft wrapping
techniques. With yarns wrapped around each other and tightly
packed, knobs were allowed to protrude on the sandal sole,
creating relief patterns. In the interest of creating beautiful
textured designs on the soles of sandals, many separate
decisions and executions were necessary.

Specialists in textile technology have subdivided sandal morphology, decoration, and manufacture to identify subtle differences in time and place of manufacture. Whether or not the unique styling of each specimen was indeed an identifying footprint for a certain individual in his or her community, the taxonomic subdivisions are going to be "footprints" for archaeologists, museum curators, and others interested in the subject to use in putting each object in its correct time and place and understanding sandals in their cultural context.

It might be asked why clothing destined to be worn on the soles of human feet—abraded between the body and the ground with every step—should receive so much creative effort and expression. A definitive answer is impossible. The human aspirations that lead to much of creative genius are based in value systems such as artistic expression, efficiency of manufacture relative to the work involved, and importance of the resulting product. Availability of materials sometimes has a bearing; yucca is a common plant in this area.

Social status is often reflected in the quality of clothing, sometimes indicating the time and labor commitment necessary to process fiber and yarn, dye the raw material, and construct the sandals. Dress may also reflect whether it was made and worn for life-passage events such as births, marriages, and deaths or merely for the routine of everyday activities. Even the most complex types of Anasazi sandals have been found worn and discarded in trash middens. Examination of cultural diversity reveals countless examples of materials and decoration reflecting the nature of people and the time in which they lived.

Suffice it to say that the Anasazi put great importance into making and decorating their footgear. Perhaps distinctive shoe prints were needed for group identification such as that of clan or tribe, or even for personal identification. Perhaps a person's sandals, when observed at the entrance of a dwelling, served notice to other arrivals as to who was inside. This signal might attract certain visitors, allow others to practice avoidance, or merely be information. Designs may have had identifying characteristics for age, sex, religious society, or tribal membership. These are conjectures. Perhaps with future studies, such correlations will be made.

Each design seems to follow certain rules of color combination and overall structure, yet the diversity of design content is so vast that it is impossible to classify the designs intuitively into groups that might correlate with human social categories. What is clear is that sandal decoration, together with the similar designs found on pottery, baskets, and other textiles, represents an artistic tradition as complicated and interesting as that of the more highly visible rock art. The two styles of design, however, could not be more different even though they persisted side by side in the same communities.

As modern observers, distanced from the Anasazi makers and wearers of these sandals by centuries, we can merely feel fortunate to have access to such creative human endeavor.

/// \\\ /// \\\ ///

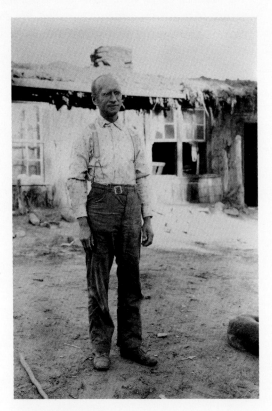

Byron Cummings at
Richard Wetherill's
trading post at Oljato

Cummings party camp
on way to Oraibi,
Arizona

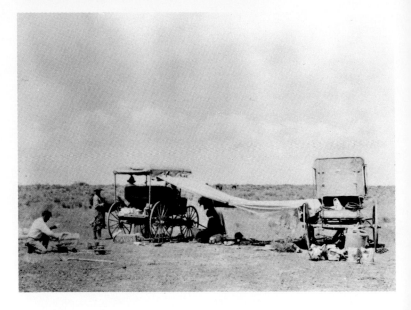

Archaeology

Duncan Metcalfe

/// \\\ /// \\\ /// \\\ /// \\\ /// \\\ /// \\\ /// \\\ /// \\\ /// \\\ /// \\\ /// \\\ /// \

A mong the Anasazi sandals illustrated in this catalog, the earliest recovered specimen appears to have come from the excavation of Alkali Ridge in 1908, and the most recent from Ivy Shelter, which was excavated in 1962. The collection therefore spans fifty-four years of archaeological investigation, or about three generations of archaeologists. During that time archaeology matured greatly as a discipline: the questions asked by archaeologists changed, and methods and techniques used in the field and in the laboratory increased in both sophistication and number. These changes, and their influence on the character of the museum's sandal collection, can be broadly outlined by considering the contributions of two archaeologists whose work resulted in the recovery of most of the sandals in this collection: Byron Cummings and Jesse D. Jennings.

Byron Cummings joined the faculty of the University of Utah in 1893 as an instructor in Latin and English. He quickly became interested in the archaeology of southern Utah and assisted in building the university's archaeological collections, established only a few years earlier. The character of Cummings's archaeological work prior to 1906 is poorly documented. In his autobiography, Cummings wrote, "In 1896 I spent the first quarter of summer session at the University of Chicago, doing graduate work in archaeology" (1953, 31). Otherwise he mentions no interest in archaeology until about 1906. After that date, the nature of his career becomes much clearer because of the writings of Neil Judd.

According to Judd, a student and nephew of Cummings's who went on to become a well-known archaeologist in his own right, Cummings's interest in the archaeology of southern Utah and northern Arizona was sparked in 1906 by a horse-and-buggy trip through Nine Mile Canyon with its spectacular ruins. With a single exception, Cummings went into the field every summer between 1907 and 1915. In the spring of 1915, after serving nine years as the first dean of the School of Arts and Sciences, Cummings and sixteen other faculty members resigned from the University of Utah in protest over faculty dismissals. That same year, he joined the faculty at the University of Arizona as professor of archaeology and director of the Arizona State

Betatakin, Arizona,
1909

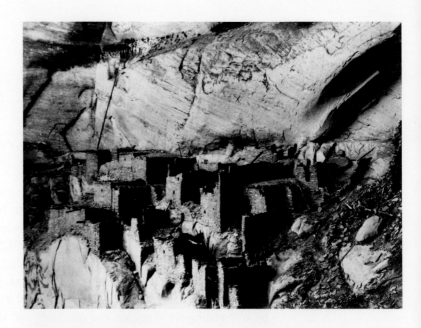

Byron Cummings at
Sega at Sosa (now
called Tsegi Hatsosie),
Arizona

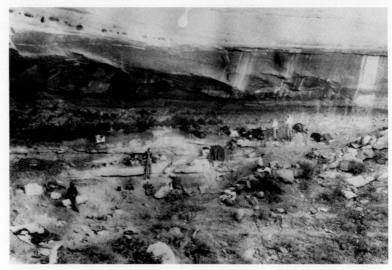

Museum. He held those positions until his retirement. He died
in 1954 at the age of 93.

Southwestern archaeology was in its infancy during the time
Cummings added to the collections of what later became the
Utah Museum of Natural History. By today's standards
Cummings's field notes are cursory, his excavation techniques
substandard, and the provenience (context of recovery) of
collected artifacts, including sandals, uncertain. This is true for
much of the archaeological work conducted before and during
Cummings's era. Most investigators were not formally trained in
archaeology, maps were crude or nonexistent, and questions
about anything other than the artifacts themselves seldom arose.
The term "Anasazi" was yet to be applied to the sites
Cummings investigated, and another twenty years would pass
between his early work and the formalization of the

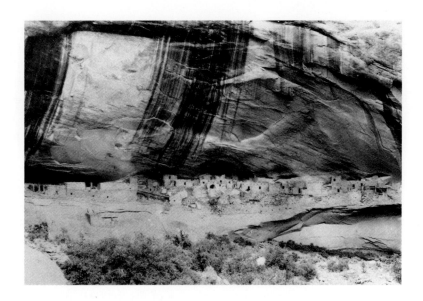

Basketmaker-Pueblo sequence that has become the standard
developmental classification for the Anasazi archaeological
complex. The era in which Cummings worked is illustrated by
Neil Judd's recollection of the beginning of the 1907 field
season.

> Overnight by train from Salt Lake City to Thompson's Spring,
> a water stop on the [Denver and Rio Grande]; thence by
> four-horse freight wagon a day and a half to the cable ferry at
> Moab; thence two more days to Monticello—the mere
> approach to our summer's work was an experience in itself.
>   At Monticello horses and mules were saddled for the trip
> down Montezuma Creek and thence to Bluff City. . . .
>   There was no auto road from Blanding to the White
> Canyon natural bridges in 1907. Indeed, there was no
> Blanding. When we camped there on our way back to
> Monticello in early September, a lone sheep herder's wagon
> parked beside a juniper proclaimed the town's beginnings.
> (Judd 1950, 13)

Studying collections such as those made by Cummings may
elicit some contradictions. When reading this catalog one can't
help but speculate about the people behind these sandals. The
obvious skill that went into their construction, the pattern of
wear on the soles, the practicality of the repairs—all are
reminders of the basic human requirements faced by all people
across all time.
    One might also speculate how much more we would know
about the people who wore these sandals if they could
somehow be "rerecovered" using modern field techniques.
Samples of the soil around the sandals could be collected and
analyzed for seeds from past meals. The surfaces of metates

could be washed with sterile water, and the pollen rinsed from their surfaces could be examined for further evidence of what was eaten. Associated projectile points could be examined for blood residue, and the type of animal blood could be determined. The point is simple: artifacts, even artifacts as unique and exquisite as those illustrated in this book, yield only a minute fraction of knowledge compared to the information that can be obtained from studying all the archaeologically associated material.

Unfortunately, artifacts can't be rerecovered. What many people don't realize is that an archaeological excavation destroys the site just as effectively as a bulldozer might. The only difference between these kinds of destructive activities lies in the careful accumulation of notes, maps, photographs, field specimen logs and, of course, the artifacts themselves. The interpretive value of the artifacts is integrally linked to the excavation documentation.

The second largest segment of the sandal collection was recovered during the Upper Colorado River Basin Archaeological Salvage Project. Jesse D. Jennings led the University of Utah's participation in this Glen Canyon project, a large, multidisciplinary project initiated in the late 1950s to identify and study prehistoric and historic sites in jeopardy of being destroyed by the construction of Glen Canyon Dam and the creation of Lake Powell. This work took place more than fifty years after Cummings first started investigating the archaeology of the Four Corners region. Because of the relative inaccessibility of Glen Canyon, the logistics of fieldwork were probably rather similar, but archaeology in the Southwest had been professionalized by this time. Maps were available for most areas, radiocarbon dating had been developed, and the forms still employed today to document excavations were already in use. Archaeology had advanced tremendously in field methods.

Jennings is a professionally trained archaeologist who received his graduate education at the University of Chicago. He came to the University of Utah in 1948 as an associate professor and curator of the Museum of Anthropology after having served nearly a decade in the National Park Service. Soon after moving to Utah, he initiated the now famous excavations of Danger Cave near Wendover, Utah, and the Statewide Archaeological Survey. The goal of the survey was to provide for the systematic study of the prehistory of the state, with emphasis on regions that were poorly known. Jennings investigated the prehistory of the Great Basin and the Colorado Plateau for the next thirty years. At this writing he is an Emeritus Distinguished Professor of Anthropology living in Oregon and still teaching on occasion at the University of Oregon.

It is considerably easier to discuss Jennings and his view of

Jesse Jennings at
Glen Canyon

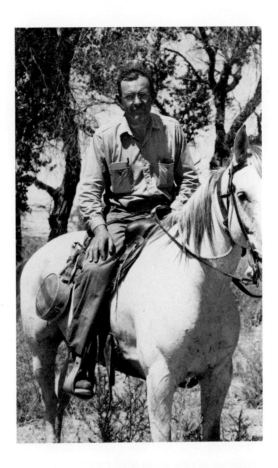

Excavation at Talus
Ruin, Glen Canyon

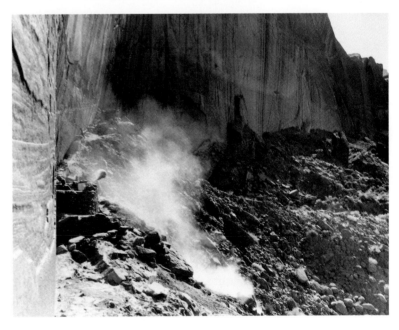

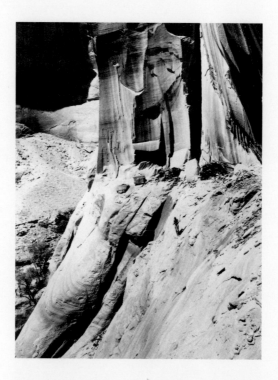

archaeology because it was through him that I initially became
truly interested in the discipline while a student in the last field
school he taught. Jennings had three basic commandments. First,
the safety and well-being of the crew was paramount. This
required preparation and careful attention, and anyone
demonstrating a lack of attention, at any level, was likely to
receive a "that's a horse on you, boy." I had four "horses" by
the end of the summer. One was for forgetting to make sure
there was film for the camera before leaving camp. The
rationale was simple. Forgetting to replace the spent film in a
camera might cost only an hour of work, but neglecting to refill
water containers or gas tanks or forgetting first-aid kits or
other essential equipment could affect the safety of the crew.
Inattention was not tolerated.

Second only to personal safety was Jennings's emphasis on
complete documentation of all archaeological investigations.
Field notes, photographs, and maps were treated as priceless, as
indeed they are, and every conceivable precaution was taken to
ensure their safety. All field notes, including the logs of
photographs taken and artifacts collected, were written in
duplicate. Whenever possible, preferably each week, the
duplicates and originals were separated and one set sent to the
university. When returning from excavations in Samoa, crew
members' flights were staggered so that the original and
duplicate notes would be on separate planes, just in case.

Last, Jennings had absolutely no tolerance for "cookbook"
archaeology. The operations manual of the Statewide
Archaeological Survey declared: "Each site is to be regarded as

unique. It must be dug on its own terms. It is the responsibility of each excavator to see that the digging techniques are appropriate, not rote or ritualized at each site" (Jennings 1969, 11). His most common admonition to students learning excavation techniques was to "use the coarsest tool for the job." If the task could be accomplished with a shovel rather than a trowel, the shovel was always preferred. Jennings also had little patience with speculation during the course of an excavation.

> Excavators are further reminded that the data, the sequence of events, and the relationships at any given site are observable. They are in the ground and must be dug for. Hours spent in setting and resetting stakes or in speculation about objects or phenomena which are not yet excavated is less rewarding than digging. Archaeology is done by moving dirt, and noting relationships and thinking about them. (Jennings 1969, 12)

Any archaeological collection that spans fifty-four years of recovery will have its share of weaknesses from a scientific perspective. It is encouraging to note, however, a recent trend that has become known as "reverse archaeology." Because of the number and importance of museum collections that were recovered under less than ideal conditions around the turn of the century, some professional and avocational archaeologists are trying to establish the archaeological origins for artifacts in those collections. Using historic photographs and diaries and discovering historic inscriptions left by early expeditions, the goal is to establish the sites from which the various artifacts came (see Atkins 1993). This sort of reverse archaeology would be very beneficial with the sandals collected by Byron Cummings in the early 1900s. Perhaps by studying notes, descriptions, and photographs, original locations in sites could be identified for many of the sandals.

Archaeologists in the future will probably never have the opportunity to recover even one sandal specimen like those shown in this catalog during their entire career. The odds are thousands to one against discovering a site with the characteristics necessary for preserving perishable artifacts for hundreds or thousands of years that hasn't been previously excavated, vandalized, or destroyed by the development of urban and rural landscapes. It is important to be able to study a collection like the one portrayed in this book to heighten awareness and understanding of the diversity and technical skill of this important aspect of Anasazi culture.

Plant Perspective

Richard Holloway   /// \\\ /// \\\ /// \\\ /// \\\ /// \\\ /// \\\ /// \\\ /// \\\ /// \\\ /// \\\ //

D ocumenting the sandal collection at the Utah Museum of Natural History required that the materials from which the sandals were constructed be identified. To accomplish this, 217 fiber samples taken from warp, weft, cordage, and padding were analyzed for fiber content.

Samples were mounted on microscope slides and examined with an aus-Jena Laboval Compound microscope. Several drops of cytoseal 280—a high-viscosity acrylic resin that produces a permanent mount—covered each fiber. After drying, the specimens were examined using 200X magnification or, occasionally, 400X magnification.

All identifications were based on comparison with modern fibers in the reference collections of either Quaternary Services or the biology department herbarium at the University of New Mexico. Virtually all the specimens examined—over 97 percent—were identified as belonging to the genus *Yucca*.

There was little difference in composition between the warp and weft samples submitted. Fibers from the weft samples, however, were generally finer and appeared softer than those from the warp. I suspect that the weft samples, although composed of the same raw materials, were worked to a greater degree in processing than were those from the warp.

The fibers of several genera of the Agavaceae have been previously examined by Bell and King (1944). These authors noted that, in general, yucca fibers are long and taper to a rounded end. They also found that fibers of the broad-leaf yuccas were very similar to each other and that fibers of the narrow-leaf species were similarly identical to each other. However, there were observable differences between the broad- and narrow-leaf groups. These differences lay primarily in the width of the lumen of the fiber. In the narrow-leaf species, the lumen was generally consistent and about as wide as the cell wall. In the broad-leaf species, the cell wall was twice the thickness of the lumen. Although some of the sandal specimens examined did not break apart readily, the characteristics of the fibers more closely resembled those of the narrow-leaf yucca group.

There is difficulty, however, in assigning these fibers to a particular group of yucca species. Yuccas as a group hybridize very readily, and taxonomists are generally conservative when assigning species identifications to anything less than the entire plant (Webber 1953).

The yucca plant is common throughout the American Southwest. As described by Correl and Johnston (1979), yucca is rather large, containing a thick, branching, mostly underground caudex (the woody base of a perennial plant). This is common in the narrow-leaf yuccas. The broad-leaf yuccas generally have a distinct woody trunk above ground. The leaves are numerous and clustered at the ends of the branches or main stem. The leaves are generally narrow (in relation to length), and either thin and flaccid (narrow-leaf) or thick and rigid (broad-leaf). These leaves are commonly spine-tipped with corneous (hornlike texture) or filiferous (threadlike or hairlike) margins. The threadlike margins are usually associated with the narrow-leaf variety, which, because of its ease of procurement, may make up the bulk of the material in the sandal collection.

Although I suspect that the narrow-leaf varieties of yucca were being used, I hesitate to assign particular species or species groups to these identifications based only upon the fibers. Thus, for the purpose of this investigation, identification stopped at the genus level.

Yucca leaves were prepared and processed in a number of ways, judging from historic accounts from several Pueblo groups (Kent 1983). Acoma and Laguna techniques involved crushing the leaves and cleaning the fibers by scraping (Swank 1932, 76). Tewa and Cochiti techniques involved either boiling or pit roasting, followed by chewing to free the fibers (Robbins, Harrington, and Freire-Marreco 1916, 50–51). Kent quotes a detailed account of the Zuni method as described by Stevenson (1915, 78–79).

The appearance of the yucca fibers evidently varied with the preparation technique. The most common technique was one in which the fibers were incompletely separated from the pulp of the yucca leaf, giving an appearance similar to those of the specimens examined during the present investigation. In Rohn's study at Mug House (1971), it was suggested that this technique may have made twisting easier because of the sticky properties of the pulp component. At least one (rare) type of yucca preparation produced "soft, fuzzy yucca that can easily be confused with cotton because of its light color" (Kent 1983, 23). While a few sandal specimens exhibited such an appearance, microscopic examination revealed that the fibers were indeed yucca.

Even at sites that have shown more diversity in weaving materials (Holloway 1991), yucca still dominates the assemblages and was the preferred material for woven sandals.

Sandal Styles, Materials, and Techniques

Kathy Kankainen   /// \\\ /// \\\ /// \\\ /// \\\ /// \\\ /// \\\ /// \\\ /// \\\ /// \\\ /// \\\ /// \\\ ///

A nasazi sandal styles varied according to the construction technique used and the preference of the weaver. Toes might be rounded, squared, tapered, pointed, or even scalloped or heart-shaped. Heels could be rounded, squared, cupped, or puckered. The original shape may now be distorted, owing to wear and the impact of time and the environment.

For the same reasons, ties and attachments in the sandal collection are usually incomplete. Remnants of ties, however, help us reconstruct the ways in which sandals were secured to the foot. Ties were made from yucca leaves, yucca cordage, or, rarely, hide strips. Sandals were attached to the foot in ways similar to those employed today, with the addition of center toe loops extending over the second and third toes. Some shapes and tie arrangments are shown in Figure 1.

Yucca leaves were the primary source of material for Anasazi sandals. Weavers used them whole, split, separated or broken down for spinning. When used in leaf form elements were predominantly left unspun, but sometimes were twisted. On the sandals shown in this catalog, the cortex (outer layer) of the leaf is usually intact unless the material was separated, in which case decortication (removal of the outer layer) might occur naturally.

Yarn or cordage was made from yucca leaves after the leaf was broken down into loose fibers by methods that included retting (soaking), pounding, shredding, boiling, freezing, chewing, and scraping. The loose fibers are drawn into a long, continuous strand by spinning. Spindles came into use around A.D. 500—but without a spindle, fibers can be rolled against the thigh with one hand while the other hand lengthens the strand as it is twisted.

To make a plied yarn or cord two or more strands are usually spun separately in one direction and then twisted together in the opposite direction. Re-plied cordage was made of two or more plied cords. Cordage was used for both passive and active elements in weaving sandals, as well as for attaching a sandal to the foot.

In the catalog descriptions, the small letter z or s denotes the direction of original spin, and the capital letter Z or S denotes the direction of twist (Figure 2). Cordage is assumed to be

Figure 1. Sandal shapes and tie arrangements.

Sandal with pointed toe, cupped heel
Sandal with scalloped toe, puckered heel
Sandal with squared toe, squared heel

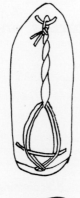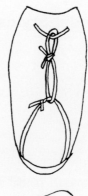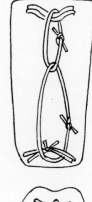

Sandal with tapered toe and jog, squared heel
Sandal with tapered toe, cupped heel
Sandal with heart-shaped toe, puckered heel

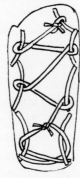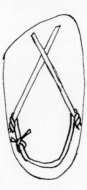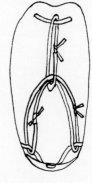

Sandal with rounded toe, rounded heel
Sandal with rounded toe, squared heel
Sandal with squared toe, cupped heel

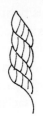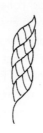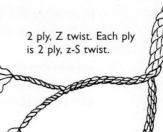

Figure 2. Cordage

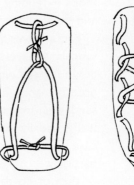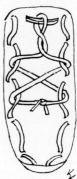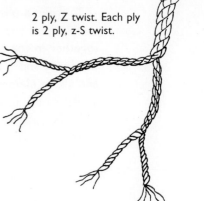

2 ply, Z twist. Each ply is 2 ply, z-S twist.

s spin or S twist   z spin or Z twist

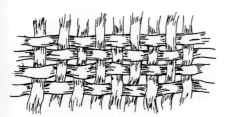

Figure 3. Balanced
plain weave

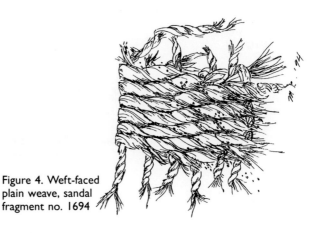

Figure 4. Weft-faced
plain weave, sandal
fragment no. 1694

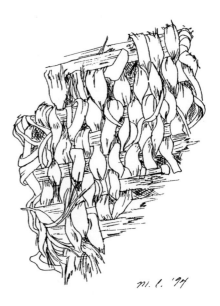

Figure 5. Warp-faced
plain weave, sandal
fragment no. 42KA443
FS13.13

decorticated—that is, the outer layer of yucca leaf has been
removed—unless stated otherwise.

Because Anasazi sandal weavers utilized the yucca plant in
different forms, ranging from the leaf itself to a highly processed,
soft, plied element, this publication uses the terms *leaf element*
and *cordage* rather than the term *yarn*.

Anasazi weavers made sandals using any of three basic
techniques: plain weave, twining, and plaiting. In *plain weave*—
the single most common technique seen in the collection,
accounting for almost half the specimens—the active
(horizontal) elements, called the *weft*, pass over and under the
passive (vertical) elements, or the *warp*. Warps and wefts
consisted either of cordage made from prepared yucca leaves or
of the yucca leaf used whole, split, or separated.

In a *balanced plain weave* (Figure 3), warp and weft are
approximately the same size and are equally visible. In a *weft-
faced plain weave* (Figure 4), wefts are packed closely together,
covering the warp. Most of the plain weave sandals in this
collection are weft faced. In the less common *warp-faced plain*

Figure 6. Plain weave
knotted starts and
finishes.

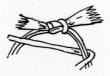

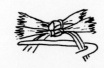

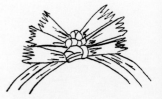

Sandal start with one
knot at toe

Sandal start with two
knots at toe

Sandal start with three
knots at toe

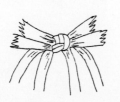

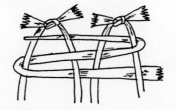

Knotted sandal starts
with four warps

Figure 7. Plain weave
wefts.

Plain-weave sandal,
fragment no. 2530

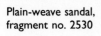

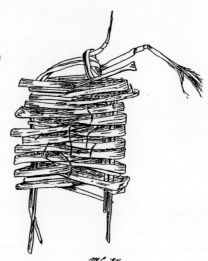

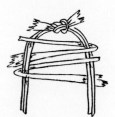

Weaving with short
wefts

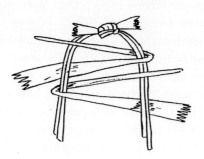

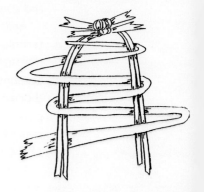

Weaving with long
wefts

Alternate tight and
loose weaving of wefts

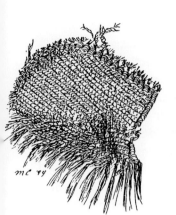

Figure 8. Twined sandal fragment, no. 2818

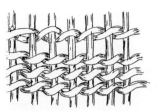

Figure 9. Simple twining with a half-turn twist

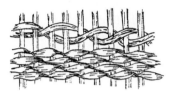

Figure 10. 2/2 alternate pair twining

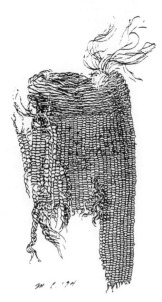

Figure 12. Fragment of sandal made in both plain weave and twining, no. 2606

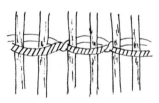

Figure 11. Twining with a full-turn twist

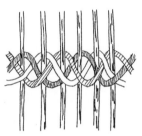

Figure 13. Three-element twining

weave (Figure 5), warps are set close together so that wefts are covered.

One type of plain weave sandal that is abundant in the collection consists of warps that are predominantly flat leaf elements tied into knots at the toe and heel. In a knotted start, two, four, six, or more warps are aligned parallel to each other and then tied into one or more knots at the toe. In a knotted finish, warps are tied together at the heel with one or more knots. The accompanying drawings illustrate these variations of knotted starts and finishes.

Figures 6 and 7 illustrate several methods of weaving a common plain weave sandal with a knotted start tying together two warps or warp units and weaving with narrow, whole yucca leaves. In one, weaving with short wefts begins with the narrow ends of the leaves on top and finishes with the wide ends on the sole, which is usually shredded for padding. If wefts are longer, their ends may extend beyond the warp edge of the sandal, increasing its width. Finally, long wefts may encircle warps alternately tightly and loosely, which extends the width of the sandal beyond the warp edge.

Unlike plain weave, a second technique, *twining* (Figure 8), accounted for only nine sandals in the collection, but is one of several techniques used in weaving composite sandals. In twined sandals, wefts work as pairs or triplets and are twisted as they pass over and under the vertical warps. In the basic technique, *simple twining* (Figure 9), wefts pass around single warps, or over one, under one (1/1). The appearance of simple twining is similar to that of plain weave when wefts are packed tightly. To keep the twist at the same slant in each row, the twist order must be reversed at the selvage edge. If the twist order is not reversed, the twining is counter to that on the adjacent row and creates a chained effect.

In *alternate pair twining* (Emery 1966), wefts pass around two warps, or over two, under two (2/2) (Figure 10), but at the edges they advance just one warp in every other row, so that the stitches alternate back and forth. The use of alternate pair twining to create a scalloped toe start is illustrated in two accompanying drawings. A third variety of twining, called *full-turn twining* (Figure 11), is generally used when twining with two colors. By incorporating a full turn between warps, one color will appear on the surface of the woven item and the other color will appear on the reverse side. The color scheme can be altered at any point by inserting a regular half-turn to reverse the color order.

Eight sandals in the collection show a combination of plain weave and twining (Figure 12). The forward one-third of the sandal is twined, usually in 2/2 alternate pair twining, and the remaining two-thirds, to the heel, is woven in plain weave. In some sandals it appears that the plain weave section has one or two rows of three-element twining (Figure 13) alternating with three to six rows of plain weave (or simple twining). This creates a ridge that appears only on the sole.

Approximately one-third of the sandals in the collection utilize the technique known as *plaiting* (Figure 14). This technique is sometimes referred to as braiding, but we prefer plaiting because it is a recognized term that is used more frequently in discussions of basketry and weaving.

In plaited sandals, all elements are active and usually close to the same size. They weave back and forth, crossing each other at set intervals, but they may incorporate shifts in interval for design change, shaping, and edge treatment. In *simple plaiting*, the elements simply pass over and under each other—they are said to be plaited at one interval. In *twill plaiting* (Figures 15 and 16), one set of elements passes over and under two or more opposite elements in a staggered fashion creating a chevron or herringbone pattern with resulting intervals of 2/2, 2/3, etc.

Forty-seven sandals in the collection is of a type we call

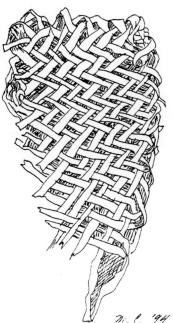

Figure 14. 2/2 twill plaiting, sandal fragment no. 2569

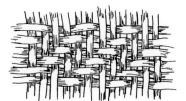

Figure 15. 2/2 twill plaiting

Figure 16. Three varieties of a plaited start, folded at the toe

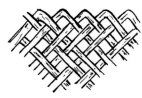

Single

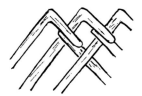

Spliced

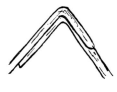

Doubled

Figure 17. Sole of a composite sandal fragment, no. 2846

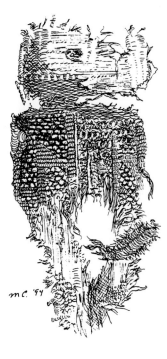

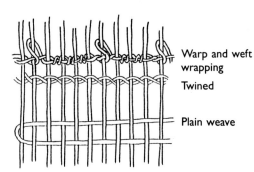

"B" weaving

"A" weaving

Figure 18. Geometric patterning technique.

Warp and weft wrapping

Twined

Plain weave

Figure 19. Geometric relief patterning technique.

Figure 20. Scalloped toe start and puckered heel finish.

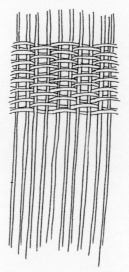

Warps are aligned parallel and wefts are woven in 2/2 alternate pair twining for a short distance.

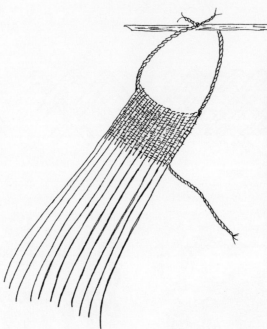

Woven section of warps is folded over a flexible element or cord that is suspended from one point. The doubled warps are woven in 2/2 alternate pair twining for the forward section of sandal. They then end or are cut, and weaving continues on single warps.

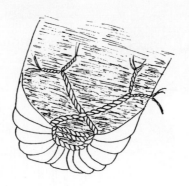

Puckered heel finish. One to three of the outer warps from each side of heel are laid across the heel, and the remaining warps wrap around this cord. Outer warps are pulled to create puckering. Heel cords can be crossed and stitched into the sandal, tied, or extended as an ankle loop.

composite (Figure 17). They are woven in plain weave or twining or both, combined with weft wrapping. Weft and warp wrapping create relief or raised areas that may be woven with dyed or natural-colored wefts in vertical or horizontal bars or complicated geometrical patterns. These composite sandals have warps, wefts, and ties of cordage. The cordage is highly processed and refined, creating a beautiful, soft, yet strong element. The finely woven, intricate composite sandals, collected predominantly in northern Arizona, represent the height of complexity in Anasazi sandals and demonstrate the genius of the weavers and their mastery of aesthetics in design.

Anasazi weavers were not always content to leave their sandals unornamented. Using dyed or natural-colored wefts, they could create a sandal or an area of a sandal with a geometric pattern or a raised design using dyed or plain elements.

A pattern could be constructed in a flat weave if two wefts of different colors were twined with a full turn so that one color showed on the upper surface and the other color showed on the sole. A half-turn was employed for color change.

To create a raised, rather than a flat, geometric pattern, diffused on the sole but sharply visible on the upper surface, a weaver carried a static weft of one color across the front of the warps while wrapping a weft of another color around warp and weft for one row. In the next row, the static weft switches to the back of the warps and the other weft wraps around the warp and weft. Geometric patterns were achieved by exchanging the color positions of the static and active wefts. Alfred V. Kidder (1926) referred to this technique as "A" and "B" weaving on the basis of an unwoven composite sandal (Figure 18).

With only one exception, raised bar patterns appeared in the collection on the soles of sandals in natural-colored wefts. Horizontal bars were constructed by wrapping wefts, and vertical bars by wrapping warps. Wrapping was done in the overall context of twining or plain weave, which acted as a binder for the wrapped rows and created a smooth, ribbed pattern on the opposite side.

When Kidder disarticulated a composite sandal in 1926, he determined that four rows were necessary for geometric relief patterns (Figure 19). One row is twined with inserts of wraps. A double wrap by one weft around the warp creates a vertical raised bar. A double wrap by the weft around the other weft creates a horizontal raised bar. By inserting two rows of plain weave and a row of 1/1 twining, the recessed portion is accomplished.

Scalloped toes and puckered heels (Figure 20) are found

predominantly in composite sandals but are also present in plain weave and twined sandals.

Because disarticulation of sandals is no longer practiced it is impossible to determine exact interlacement of some tightly woven sandals. Replication has been experimented with but there are still mysteries in structure that evoke a continuation of study.

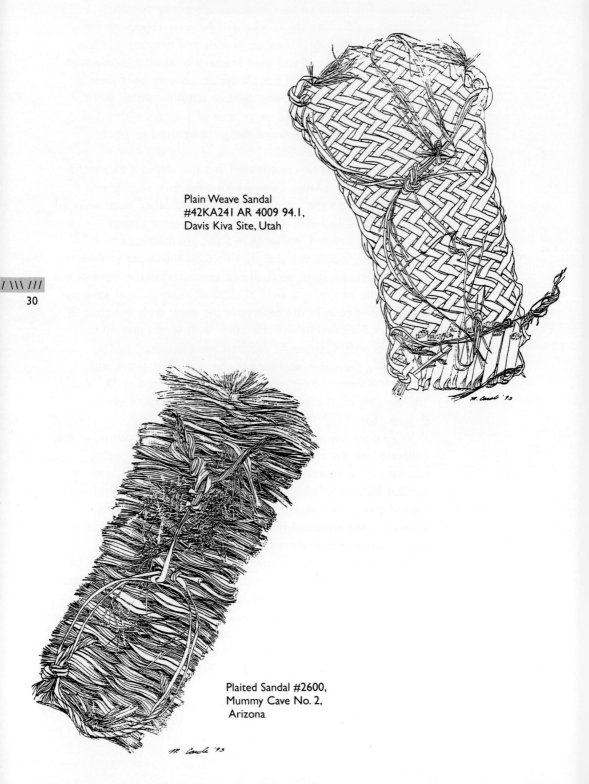

Plain Weave Sandal
#42KA241 AR 4009 94.1,
Davis Kiva Site, Utah

Plaited Sandal #2600,
Mummy Cave No. 2,
Arizona

The Catalog

/// \\\ /// \\\ /// \\\ /// \\\ /// \\\ /// \\\ /// \\\ /// \\\ /// \\\ /// \\\ /// \\\ /// \\\ ///

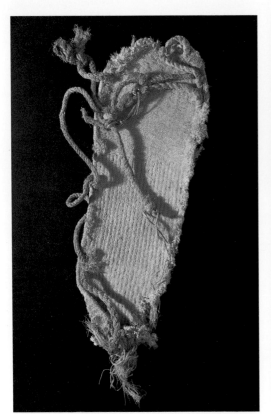

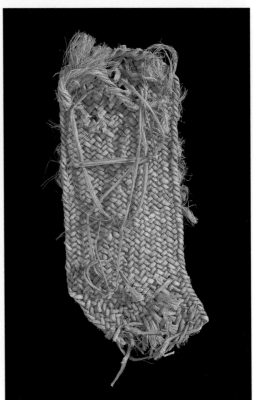

Catalog no.: AR328 85.1
Site: Alkali Ridge, Utah
Collector and date: Probably Byron Cummings,
  during Wall Expedition, 1908
Cultural period: Unknown
Construction technique: Twined
Dimensions: Length 29.0 cm, width 10.0 cm, depth
  0.97 cm
Active elements: Cordage, 2 ply, s-Z twist
Average width: 0.11 cm
Passive elements: Cordage, 3 ply, s-Z twist
Number of passive units: 25
Number in unit: 1 (except where doubled at toe)
Average width: 0.19 cm
Ties, loops, attachments: Toe: Cordage, 2 ply, Z twist
  (each ply 2 ply, z-S twist). Heel: Cordage, 7 ply.
  Edge: cordage loops, 3 ply, Z twist (each ply 2
  ply, z-S twist)
Shape: Left(?) foot shaping, scalloped toe and
  puckered heel
Start: Scalloped toe start
Body: 2/2 alternate pair twining on doubled
  elements at toe. At instep warp ends are
  truncated. Remainder of sandal appears to be
  3-4 rows of twining followed by a three-element
  twining row. Instep toward heel has two rows of
  three-element twining for approximately 9
  patterns, and then switches to one row. This
  gives a ridge pattern on sole only.
Finish: Puckered heel finish. Heel cords knot
  together, left side extends to edge loop, right
  side is broken.
Other: Mends on toe and edging loops with knotted
  leaf element

Catalog no.: AR372 86.1
Site: Alkali Ridge, Utah
Collector and date: Probably Byron Cummings
  Collection during Wall Expedition, 1908
Cultural period: Unknown
Construction technique: Plaited
Dimensions: Length 26.5 cm, width 11.0 cm, depth
  0.42 cm
Active elements: Leaf element unspun, cortex intact
Average width: 0.38 cm
Passive elements: N/A
Ties, loops, attachments: Toe: Loop of leaf element
  twisted S anchored by weaving end for a short
  distance with active element. Loop attaches to
  instep loop and heel loop. Heel: Loop of leaf
  element twisted S
Shape: Right foot shaping, disarticulated tapered toe
  and rounded heel
Start: Active elements folded at toe
Body: 2/2 twill plaiting with shifts at selvage of
  2/1/2, 2/1/2. Exhausted ends left frayed on sole
Finish: Active ends folded into sandal at heel
Other: Structural padding on sole

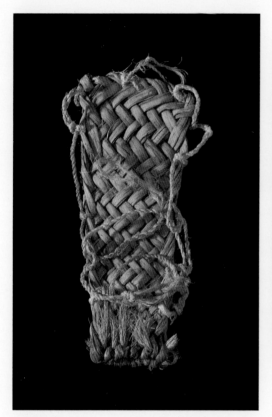
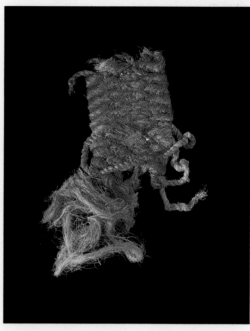

Catalog no.: 2566
Site: Baby Mummy Cave, Arizona
Collector and date: Byron Cummings, University of
   Utah Expedition, 1914
Cultural period: Unknown
Construction technique: Plaited
Dimensions: Length 23.0 cm, width 10.0 cm, depth
   0.9 cm
Active elements: Leaf element unspun, cortex intact
Average width: 0.75 cm
Passive elements: N/A
Ties, loops, attachments: Toe: Cordage 2-ply, s-Z
   twist, looped through a plaited element and
   secured with a knot. Edge: Two ply cordage, s-Z
   twist; looped along edges by encircling an active
   element and knotted. Heel: Thick heel cord
   loops across heel. Composed of two, 3 ply
   cords, twisted Z (each cord z-S twist)
Shape: Right foot shaping, squared heel and toe
Start: Eight double overlayed elements folded at
   toe forming 16 elements. After the fold, the
   initial plaiting row is over/under three.
Body: 2/2 twill plaiting for length of sandal using
   doubled elements
Finish: Leaf element folded across heel forming two
   bars and secured at one end by a knot. The
   plaiting elements are folded over the upper and
   lower bars in a pattern of every-other-one, the
   ends of one group being brought to the surface,
   the others to the reverse side. All ends are
   clipped.
Other: Possible mends at toe and edge

Catalog no.: 2567
Site: Baby Mummy Cave, Arizona
Collector and date: Byron Cummings, University of
   Utah Expedition, 1914
Cultural period: Pueblo II
Construction technique: Plain weave
Dimensions: Length 11.78 cm, width 7.00 cm, depth
   1.21 cm
Active elements: Shredded leaf element,
   decorticated, twisted S and Z
Average width: 0.73 cm
Passive elements: Cordage, element, 2 ply, s-Z twist
Number of passive units: 4
Number in unit: 1
Average width: 0.33 cm
Ties, loops, attachments: Edge: Continuous cord
   from side to side formed by cordage wrapped
   around outside warps and twisted back onto
   itself. A second cord is joined in the same
   manner on one side but broken from the
   opposite side.
Shape: Unknown; fragmentary piece
Start: Missing
Body: Tightly packed plain weave continues to heel.
   Shredded yucca weft has been gathered together
   for appropriate width of weft and twisted as it is
   woven. This gives an "S" twist in one direction
   and a "Z" twist in the opposite direction.
Finish: Missing

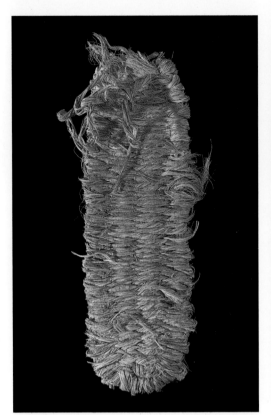

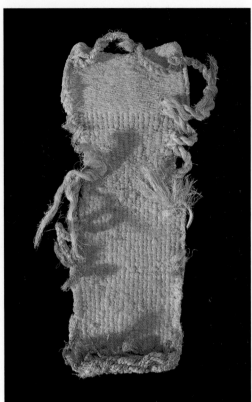

Catalog no.: 2578
Site: Baby Mummy Cave, Arizona
Collector and date: Byron Cummings, University of
   Utah Expedition, 1914
Cultural period: Unknown
Construction technique: Plain weave
Dimensions: Length 27.20 cm, width 8.66 cm, depth
   0.84 cm
Active elements: Separated leaf elements, cortex
   intact. Loosely twisted S
Average width: 0.48 cm
Passive elements: Leaf elements unspun, cortex
   intact
Number of passive units: 4
Number in unit: 2
Average width: 0.51 cm
Ties, loops, attachments: Heel: Two leaf elements
   loosely twisted S extend from both sides of heel.
   Left side tie stitches back into body of sandal.
   Edge: One leaf element from the right edge
   extends toward heel looping through both heel
   elements.
Shape: Rounded toe and squared heel
Start: Two warp units fold at toe forming two
   outside warps. Two remaining warp units lie
   folded separately, and parallel inside outer warp
   fold. After wrapping outer warp unit at toe,
   inner folded warps are stitched at fold to outer
   warp.
Body: Over-under plain weave from toe to heel
Finish: At heel warps appear knotted together in
   four (?) knots. The resulting ends of two outside
   knots are also knotted together.
Other: Structural padding on sole

Catalog no.: 2573
Site: Baby Mummy Cave, Arizona
Collector and date: Byron Cummings, University of
   Utah Expedition, 1914
Cultural period: Unknown
Construction technique: Plain weave and twined
Dimensions: Length 26.5 cm, width 11.0 cm, depth
   0.65 cm
Active elements: Cordage, 2 ply, s-Z twist
Average width: 0.13 cm
Passive elements: Cordage, 2 ply, s-Z twist
Number of passive units: 24
Number in unit: 1 (except where doubled at toe)
Average width: 0.25 cm
Ties, loops, attachments: Toe and edge: Cordage, ties
   2 ply, s-Z twist, looped and stitched into body of
   sandal and down both edges. Heel: cordage, 2
   ply, S twist, each ply made up of two warp
   element (s-Z twist)
Shape: Scalloped toe and squared heel
Start: Scalloped toe start
Body: 2/2 alternate pair twining over doubled warps
   at toe. Instep section appears different from rest
   of sandal. Could be 1/1 simple twining only.
   Lower half of sandal to heel appears to be
   woven with several (3?) rows of plain weave and
   a row of 3 element twining which gives the faint
   ridge appearance on sole. Extreme wear on sole
Finish: At heel approximately four warps are
   brought from each side and twisted together.
   Remaining warps are knotted into heel.

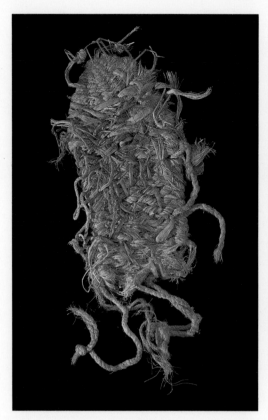

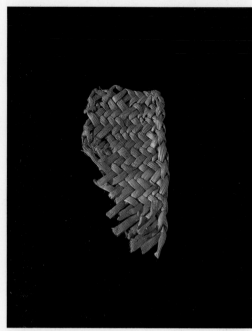

vertical and horizontal. Stitching holds desiccated heel together.

36 *Catalog no.:* 2576
Site: Baby Mummy Cave, Arizona
Collector and date: Byron Cummings, University of Utah Expedition, 1914
Cultural period: Pueblo II
Construction technique: Plain weave
Dimensions: Length 21.0 cm, width 10.5 cm, depth 1.25 cm
Active elements: Shredded leaf element, cortex intact, twisted S and Z
Average width: 0.54 cm
Passive elements: Cordage, element, 2 ply s-Z twist
Number of passive units: 6
Number in unit: 1
Average width: 0.37 cm
Ties, loops, attachments: Toe: Loop of leaf element tied to 2 ply s-Z twist cordage fragment. Heel: Cordage, 2 ply s-Z twist. One cord knotted to loop on right side. One cord knotted to a loose tie. Edge: One leaf element tie; three cordage types: all 2 ply s-Z twist but very fine, fine and coarse
Shape: Pointed toe and squared heel
Start: Three cordage warps folded at toe (one inside the other) to form six warp elements. Finer active weft elements used at start to draw into pointed toe shape
Body: Tightly packed plain weave continues to heel. Shredded yucca weft has been gathered together for appropriate width of weft and twisted as it is woven. This gives an "S" twist in one direction and a "Z" twist in the opposite direction.
Finish: Heel warps incomplete
Other: Stitching appears to be mends and runs

Catalog no.: 2569
Site: Baby Mummy Cave, Arizona
Collector and date: Byron Cummings, University of Utah Expedition, 1914
Cultural period: Unknown
Construction technique: Plaited
Dimensions: Length 15.50 cm, width 8.60 cm, depth 0.50 cm
Active elements: Leaf element unspun, cortex intact
Average width: 0.53 cm
Passive elements: N/A
Ties, loops, attachments: None apparent
Shape: Unknown, fragmentary
Start: Nine leaf elements are folded at toe to make 18 active elements.
Body: 2/2 twill plaiting for length of fragment
Finish: Missing

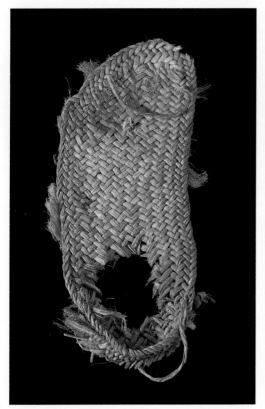
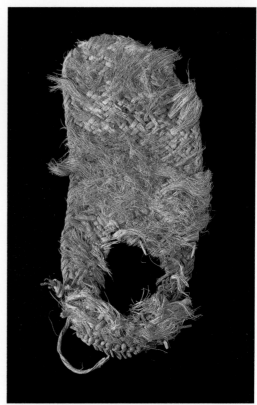

Catalog no.: 2575
Site: Baby Mummy Cave, Arizona
Collector and date: Byron Cummings, University of
    Utah Expedition, 1914
Cultural period: Unknown
Construction technique: Plaited
Dimensions: Length 25.98 cm, width 11.04 cm,
    depth 0.66 cm
Active elements: Leaf element unspun, cortex intact
Average width: 0.49 cm
Passive elements: N/A
Ties, loops, attachments: Toe: Leaf element tie,
    twisted S. Heel: Leaf element tie twisted loops
    across heel.
Shape: Left foot shaping, round tapered toe with a
    jog, round cupped heel
Start: Approximately 10 elements are folded at toe
    to make 20 active elements. Another element is
    folded and added at toe jog.
Body: 2/2 twill plaiting with 2/3/2 at edges which
    are pulled tight. Exhausted wide ends are left
    shredded on sole.
Finish: At heel weaving is pulled tight. Half of the
    ends are left protruding on reverse and the
    other half are knotted around adjacent elements.
Other: Structural padding on sole

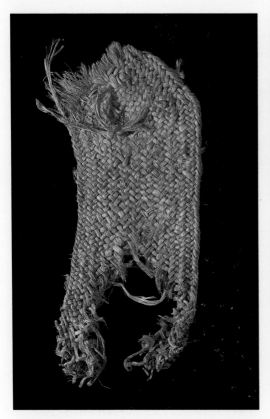 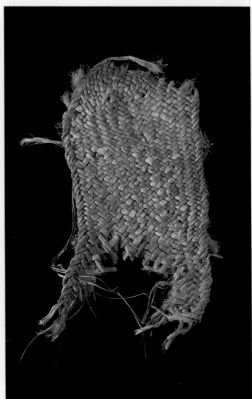

38 *Catalog no.:* 2587
Site: Baby Mummy Cave, Arizona
Collector and date: Byron Cummings, University of
   Utah Expedition, 1914
Cultural period: Unknown
Construction technique: Plaited
Dimensions: Length 26.5 cm, width 11.0 cm, depth
   0.64 cm
Active elements: Leaf element unspun, cortex intact
Average width: 0.34 cm
Passive elements: N/A
Ties, loops, attachments: Toe: Shredded leaf element
   looped through sandal and knotted at toe
Shape: Right foot shaping, tapered toe with jog,
   heel missing
Start: Active elements folded at toe. An additional
   active element is folded at toe jog.
Body: 2/2 twill plaiting with some shifts to facilitate
   shaping. Edges plaited 2/3/2 and drawn in tightly.
   Heel also appears drawn in. Exhausted wide
   ends left frayed on sole
Finish: Missing
Other: Structural padding on sole

Catalog no.: 2588
Site: Baby Mummy Cave, Arizona
Collector and date: Byron Cummings, University of
   Utah Expedition, 1914
Cultural period: Unknown
Construction technique: Plaited
Dimensions: Length 23.75 cm, width 11.02 cm,
   depth 1.00 cm
Active elements: Leaf element unspun, cortex intact
Average width: 0.34 cm
Passive elements: N/A
Ties, loops, attachments: Toe: Knot remnant on sole.
   Edge, leaf ties near heel
Shape: Left foot shaping, rounded toe with jog, heel
   missing
Start: Active elements appear folded at toe.
   Element added at toe jog
Body: 2/2 twill plaiting with shifts of 3/1/2 in toe
   area, 3/2/2 at edges, and a few 2/1/2 toward
   heel. Edges are pulled in tightly. Exhausted wide
   ends are left shredded on sole.
Finish: Missing
Other: Structural padding on sole

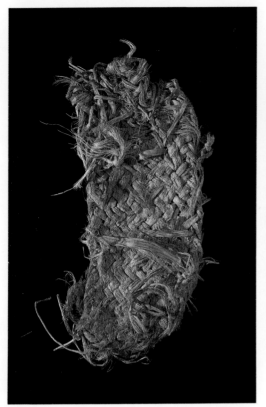

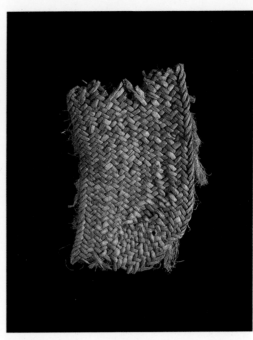

Catalog no.: 2593
Site: Baby Mummy Cave, Arizona
Collector and date: Byron Cummings, University of
  Utah Expedition, 1914
Cultural period: Unknown
Construction technique: Plaited
Dimensions: Length 23.0 cm, width 11.0 cm, depth
  0.63 cm
Active elements: Leaf element unspun, cortex intact
Average width: 0.62 cm
Passive elements: N/A
Ties, loops, attachments: Remnants of leaf element
  knots and ties appear on toe, heel and edge.
Shape: Right foot shaping, rounded heel
Start: Elements appear folded at toe.
Body: 2/2 twill plaiting with a shift of one element
  each edge of instep 2/3/2. Heel woven tightly
Finish: Active elements are wrapped and left with
  short protrusions on upper side of sandal.
Other: Mending in toe area

Catalog no.: 2603
Site: Baby Mummy Cave, Arizona
Collector and date: Byron Cummings, University of
  Utah Expedition, 1914
Cultural period: Unknown
Construction technique: Plaited
Dimensions: Length 15.5 cm, width 9.5 cm, depth
  0.86 cm
Active elements: Leaf element unspun, cortex intact
Average width: 0.37 cm
Passive elements: N/A
Ties, loops, attachments: None apparent
Shape: Left(?) foot shaping, toe jog, heel missing
Start: Missing
Body: 2/2 twill plaiting with some shifts in toe area
  for shaping and 2/3/2 on edges which are pulled
  tight. Exhausted wide ends left frayed on sole
Finish: Missing
Other: Structural padding on sole

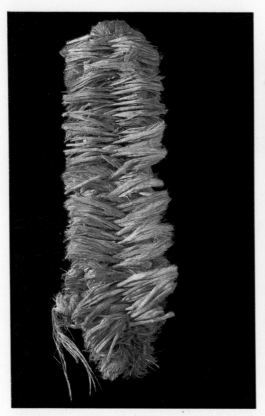

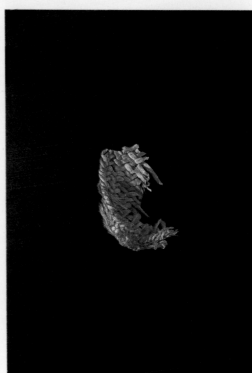

40 *Catalog no.:* 1135.1
Site: Batwoman House, Arizona
Collector and date: Byron Cummings, University of Utah Expedition, 1912
Cultural period: Pueblo III
Construction technique: Plain weave
Dimensions: Length 30 cm, width 9.2 cm, depth 2.3 cm
Active elements: Leaf element unspun, cortex intact
Average width: 0.35 cm
Passive elements: Leaf element unspun, cortex intact
Number of passive units: 2
Number in unit: 3
Average width: 0.64 cm
Ties, loops, attachments: Toe: Fragmentary leaf element tie joined to sandal on one side by a knot
Shape: Pointed toe and rounded heel
Start: Three individual leaf warps in each of two units are tied together in three separate square knots.
Body: Plain weave beginning with narrow ends of leaf element on top and ending with shredded wide ends on sole for padding
Finish: Warp ends secured by a large wrapped knot
Other: Structural padding on sole. Some of weft leaf elements have been extended directly forward from toe end simulating a toe-type padding.

Catalog no.: 1158
Site: Batwoman House, Arizona
Collector and date: Byron Cummings, University of Utah Expedition, 1912
Cultural period: Pueblo III
Construction technique: Plaited
Dimensions: Length 8.3 cm, width 5.8 cm, depth 0.60 cm
Active elements: Leaf element unspun, cortex intact
Average width: 0.41 cm
Passive elements: N/A
Ties, loops, attachments: Small leaf element extends from selvage.
Shape: Unknown, fragmentary
Start: Unknown
Body: 2/2 twill plaiting with shifts of 3/3 at selvage and 2/1/2 to shape end of sandal. Exhausted elements left long on sole and frayed
Finish: At heel half of the active elements are wrapped over a transverse rod. The other half of the elements appear wrapped around ends protruding from the first half.
Other: Structural padding on sole

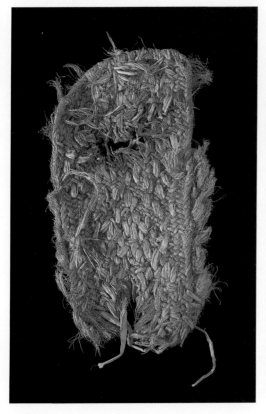

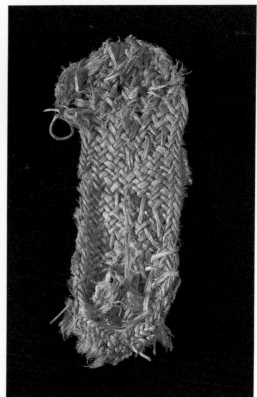

Catalog no.: 1168

Site: Batwoman House, Arizona

Collector and date: Byron Cummings, University of
Utah Expedition, 1912

Cultural period: Pueblo III

Construction technique: Plaited

Dimensions: Length 25.5 cm, width 12.0 cm, depth
1.28 cm

Active elements: Leaf element unspun, cortex intact

Average width: 0.40 cm

Passive elements: N/A

Ties, loops, attachments: Toe: Leaf element looped
and stitched across left side of toe. Edge: Leaf
element loop on left side. Remnant tie on right
side

Shape: Right foot shaping, slightly rounded toe, heel
missing

Start: Active elements folded(?) at toe

Body: 2/2 twill plaiting pulled tighter on edges.
Shifts not visible due to stitching. Exhausted ends
of elements frayed on sole

Finish: Missing

Other: Leaf elements stitched through plaited sole
with ends left frayed on sole for padding. Toe
mended or stabilized by wrapping

Catalog no.: 1170

Site: Batwoman House, Arizona

Collector and date: Byron Cummings, University of
Utah Expedition, 1912

Cultural period: Pueblo III

Construction technique: Plaited

Dimensions: Length 25.4 cm, width 12.5 cm, depth
0.95 cm

Active elements: Leaf element unspun, cortex intact

Average width: 0.38 cm

Passive elements: N/A

Ties, loops, attachments: Heel: Cordage 2 ply, s-Z
twist extends from left side of heel.

Shape: Rounded toe and cupped heel

Start: Active elements folded at toe

Body: 2/2 twill plaiting to heel where shift of
2/2/1/1/2/2 and termination of some elements
pulls selvage tightly to cup heel. Exhausted wefts
are left frayed on sole.

Finish: At heel elements are pulled tight to form
cupped heel. Elements end by wrapping and
protruding on sole.

Other: Structural padding on sole. Mending stitches
around toe and down body of sandal

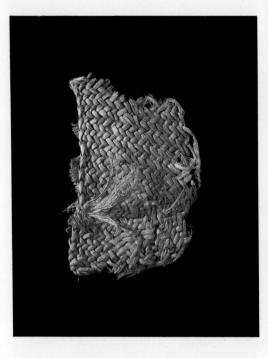

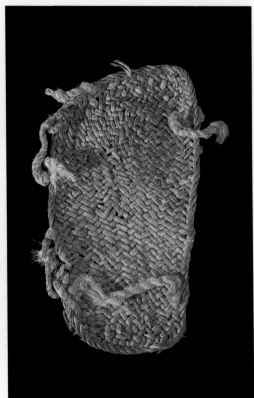

42 *Catalog no.:* 1710
Site: Batwoman House, Arizona
Collector and date: Byron Cummings, University of
   Utah Expedition, 1913
Cultural period: Pueblo III
Construction technique: Plaited
Dimensions: Length 15.0 cm, width 10.0 cm, depth
   0.93 cm
Active elements: Leaf element unspun, cortex intact
Average width: 0.88 cm
Passive elements: N/A
Ties, loops, attachments: Toe: Remnant of one
   attachment
Shape: Left(?) foot shaping
Start: Folding evident at two corners of toe; worn
   across toe
Body: 2/2 twill plaiting for length of fragment. Semi-
   circular pattern developed on one side in toe
   area. Shift patterns of 1/1 and 2/1 accommodate
   this curvature. Other attributes at the apex of
   this curve are a two-element fold facing a one-
   element fold with all elements pulled to reverse
   side.
Finish: Missing
Other: Structural padding on reverse side,
   carbonization

Catalog no.: 2801
Site: Batwoman House, Arizona
Collector and date: Byron Cummings, University of
   Utah Expedition, 1909
Cultural period: Pueblo III
Construction technique: Plaited
Dimensions: Length 24.5 cm, width 12.8 cm, depth
   0.62 cm
Active elements: Leaf element unspun, cortex intact
Average width: 0.37 cm
Passive elements: N/A
Ties, loops, attachments: Ties are cordage 2 ply, s-Z
   twist. Remnants at toe edges, heel and left side
Shape: Left foot shaping. Tapered toe with jog and
   rounded heel
Start: Active elements folded at toe. Elements
   added as necessary for tapering and toe jog
Body: 2/2 twill plaiting with a shift in toe area for
   shaping of 2/3/2. Several elements are dropped
   for shaping. Edges pulled tight with a 2/3/2 for
   raised edges
Finish: At heel ends are folded back into body of
   sandal and are left protruding on sole.
Other: Stitching is evident across heel area and toe.

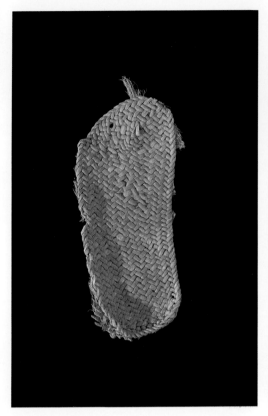

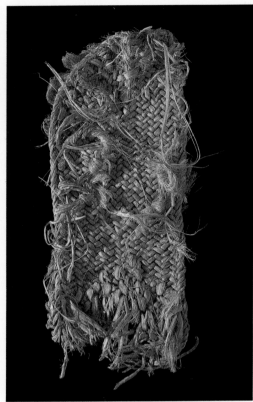

Catalog no.: 2802
Site: Batwoman House, Arizona
Collector and date: Byron Cummings, University of
    Utah Expedition, 1909
Cultural period: Pueblo III
Construction technique: Plaited
Dimensions: Length 20.0 cm, width 9.0 cm, depth
    0.62 cm
Active elements: Leaf element unspun, cortex intact
Average width: 0.37 cm
Passive elements: N/A
Ties, loops, attachments: Toe: Small leaf element
    protrudes from a hole punched (with small awl?)
    in toe area. One other hole exists at toe. Heel:
    Two awl(?) holes
Shape: Left foot shaping, rounded toe with jog and
    rounded heel
Start: Active elements folded at toe. Additional
    element folded for toe jog
Body: 2/2 twill plaiting except near toe area and ball
    of foot where irregular shifts occur. Exhausted
    ends of elements frayed on sole
Finish: At heel it appears there is a row of twining
    before heel is finished.
Other: Structural padding on sole

Catalog no.: 2803
Site: Batwoman House, Arizona
Collector and date: Byron Cummings, University of
    Utah Expedition, 1909
Cultural period: Pueblo III
Construction technique: Plaited
Dimensions: Length 26.5 cm, width 10.5 cm, depth
    0.89 cm
Active elements: Leaf element unspun, cortex intact
Average width: 0.35 cm
Passive elements: N/A
Ties, loops, attachments: Toe: Leaf elements knotted
    in loop. Edge: Right side leaf element ties
    knotted. Left side leaf elements twisted S, loop
    and stitch along edge.
Shape: Left foot shaping, rounded toe, heel missing
Start: Active elements folded at toe
Body: 2/2 twill plaiting with shifts in irregular
    pattern for shaping toe and edges of 2/3/1/3/2.
    Exhausted ends left frayed on sole
Finish: Missing, except at left edge there is a slight
    curve where elements are pulled tight
Other: Mends or reinforcement at toe and heel.
    Structural padding on sole

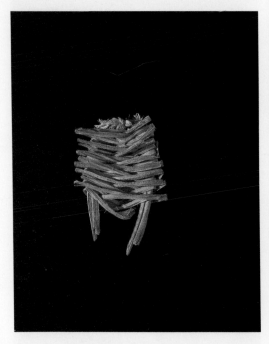
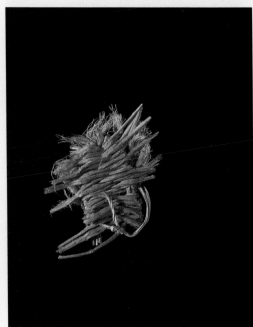

Catalog no.: 2805
Site: Batwoman House, Arizona
Collector and date: Byron Cummings, University of
    Utah Expedition, 1909
Cultural period: Pueblo III
Construction technique: Plain weave
Dimensions: Length 9.0 cm, width 10.0 cm, depth
    1.2 cm
Active elements: Leaf element unspun, cortex intact
Average width: 0.43 cm
Passive elements: Leaf element unspun, cortex intact
Number of passive units: 2
Number in unit: 1
Average width: 0.69 cm
Ties, loops, attachments: One loop around body;
    ends tied together to form loop on surface
Shape: One end slightly rounded, other end missing
Start or Finish: Warps are knotted together in one
    knot at toe.
Body: Over-under plain weave beginning with
    narrow leaves on top and ending with shredded
    wide ends on sole for padding. Ends extend
    beyond body of sandal.
Other: Structural padding on sole

44   Catalog no.: 2804
      Site: Batwoman House, Arizona
      Collector and date: Byron Cummings, University of
          Utah Expedition, 1909
      Cultural period: Pueblo III
      Construction technique: Plain weave
      Dimensions: Length 10.8 cm, width 7.0 cm, depth
          1.33 cm
      Active elements: Leaf element unspun, cortex intact
      Average width: 0.41 cm
      Passive elements: Leaf element unspun, cortex intact
      Number of passive units: 2
      Number in unit: 3
      Average width: 0.77 cm
      Ties, loops, attachments: None apparent
      Shape: Rounded end, other end missing
      Start or Finish: Warps are knotted together in two
          knots at toe.
      Body: Over-under plain weave beginning with
          narrow leaves on top and ending with shredded
          wide ends on sole for padding
      Other: Structural padding on sole

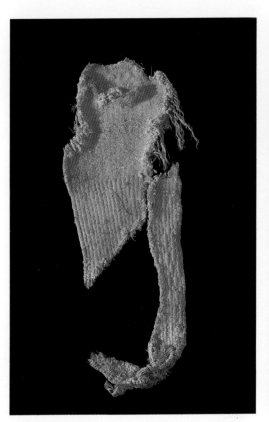

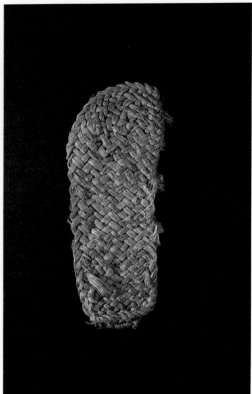

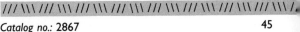

Catalog no.: 2845
Site: Batwoman House, Arizona
Collector and date: Byron Cummings, University of
  Utah Expedition, 1909
Cultural period: Basketmaker III
Construction technique: Composite
Dimensions: Length 25.54 cm, width 8.89 cm, depth
  0.79 cm
Active elements: Cordage, 2 ply, z-S twist
Average width: 0.05 cm
Passive elements: Cordage, 3 ply, z-S twist
Number of passive units: 24
Number in unit: 1 (except where doubled at toe)
Average width: 0.16 cm
Ties, loops, attachments: Toe: Cordage, remnants 3
  ply, s-Z twist. Heel: Cords formed by warps
  pulled into pucker and then pushed through
  sandal, 3 ply z twist (each ply 2 ply, z-S twist)
Shape: Scalloped toe and puckered heel
Start: Scalloped toe start
Body: 2/2 alternate pair twining over doubled warps
  for forward one-third section of sandal at which
  point doubled warps end. Remaining length of
  sandal to heel woven in raised geometric
  pattern.
Finish: Puckered heel finish. Heel cords are tucked
  into sandal.

Catalog no.: 2867
Site: Batwoman House, Arizona
Collector and date: Byron Cummings, University of
  Utah Expedition, 1912
Cultural period: Pueblo III
Construction technique: Plaited
Dimensions: Length 19.0 cm, width 7.7 cm, depth
  0.80 cm
Active elements: Leaf element unspun, cortex intact
Average width: 0.45 cm
Passive elements: N/A
Ties, loops, attachments: Edge: Remnants of leaf
  element edge loops
Shape: Left foot shaping, rounded toe and heel
Start: Active elements folded at toe
Body: 2/2 plaiting with shifts of 2/1/2 and 2/3/2 near
  toe
Finish: At heel there are two rows of wrapping with
  ends protruding on sole.
Other: Structural padding on sole

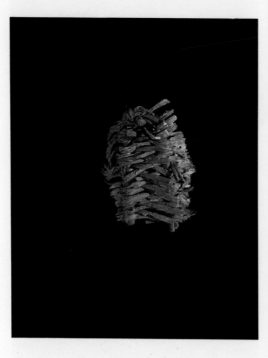

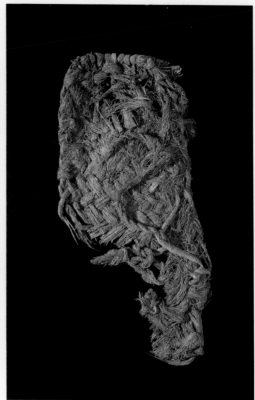

Catalog no.: 5058
Site: Batwoman House, Arizona
Collector and date: Byron Cummings, University of
   Utah Expedition, 1909
Cultural period: Pueblo III
Construction technique: Plain weave
Dimensions: Length 9.57 cm, width 7.06 cm, depth
   1.5 cm
Active elements: Leaf element unspun, cortex intact
Average width: 0.45 cm
Passive elements: Leaf element unspun, cortex intact
Number of passive units: 2
Number in unit: 1
Average width: 0.55 cm
Ties, loops, attachments: None apparent
Shape: Rounded end, other end missing
Start or Finish: Warps are knotted together in one
   knot.
Body: Over-under plain weave beginning with
   narrow leaves on top and ending with shredded
   wide ends on sole for padding
Other: Structural padding on sole

Catalog no.: 42KA433 (58.1) 23904
Site: Benchmark Cave, Utah
Collector and date: UCRBASP, 1958
Cultural period: Pueblo III
Construction technique: Plaited
Dimensions: Length 24.0 cm, width 11.5 cm, depth
   1.3 cm
Active elements: Leaf element unspun, cortex intact
Average width: 0.76 cm
Passive elements: N/A
Ties, loops, attachments: Heel: Fine weight cordage 2
   ply, s-Z twist is attached near heel. Edge:
   Cordage 2 ply s-Z twist is threaded through one
   of leaf element edge loops and square knotted
   to another cordage remnant.
Shape: Toe missing, heel rounded
Start: Missing
Body: 2/2 twill plaiting for length of sandal. No
   shifts observed. Running stitches appear
   structural.
Finish: At heel an element is brought across sandal
   from one edge. Active elements loop around this
   element with ends left protruding on sole.
   Transverse element is knotted at end.

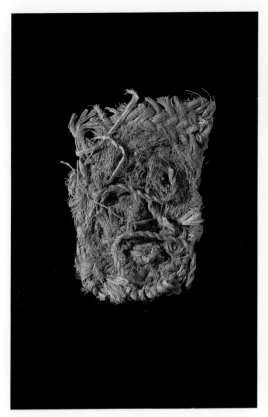 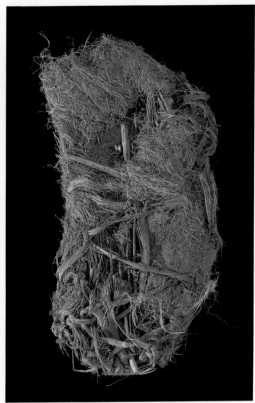

Catalog no.: 42KA433 (58.3) 23904
Site: Benchmark Cave, Utah
Collector and date: UCRBASP, 1958
Cultural period: Pueblo III
Construction technique: Plaited
Dimensions: Length 16.5 cm, width 12.2 cm, depth 1.4 cm
Active elements: Leaf element unspun, cortex intact
Average width: 0.68 cm
Passive elements: N/A
Ties, loops, attachments: Heel: Cordage 2 ply, s-Z twist lies loose on surface. Whole yucca leaf protruding on upper surface is knotted on sole. Several loose fiber knots. Edge: Leaf element looped through one edge and knotted
Shape: Toe missing, heel rounded
Start: Missing
Body: 2/2 twill plaiting for length of sandal. No shifts observed on surface but one long stitch on sole
Finish: At heel an element is brought across sandal from one edge. Active elements loop around this element with ends left protruding on sole. Transverse element is knotted at end.

Catalog no.: 42KA433 (FS35.1) 23904
Site: Benchmark Cave, Utah
Collector and date: UCRBASP, 1958
Cultural period: Pueblo II-Pueblo III
Construction technique: Plain weave
Dimensions: Length 27.0 cm, width 13.0 cm, depth 2.5 cm
Active elements: Leaf element unspun, cortex intact
Average width: 0.51 cm
Passive elements: Leaf element unspun, cortex intact
Number of passive units: 12
Number in unit: 1
Average width: 0.38 cm
Ties, loops, attachments: Toe: Leaf element ties emerge from both sides of toe. Edge: Leaf element ties lace across toe and instep area, knotted at intervals.
Shape: Left foot shaping, rounded toe, some of heel missing
Start: Six leaf elements are folded at toe over first weft element to form 12 warps.
Body: Over-under plain weave for length of sandal in approximately an even 50/50 weave structure
Finish: Missing
Other: Padding added to top of sandal

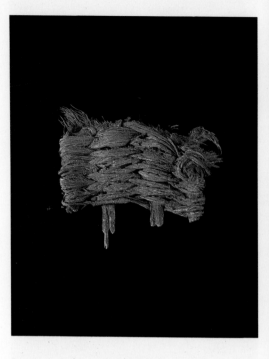

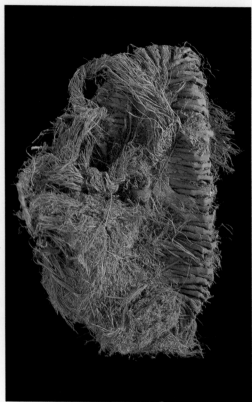

Catalog no.: 42KA433 (FS49.14) 23904
Site: Benchmark Cave, Utah
Collector and date: UCRBASP, 1958
Cultural period: Pueblo II-Pueblo III
Construction technique: Plain weave
Dimensions: Length 10.0 cm, width 11.0 cm, depth
    1.6 cm
Active elements: Leaf element unspun, cortex intact
Average width: 0.60 cm
Passive elements: Leaf element unspun, cortex intact
Number of passive units: 4
Number in unit: 1
Average width: 0.95
Ties, loops, attachments: None apparent
Shape: Fragment with one end nearly complete
Start or Finish: Two warp knots remain attached,
    one knot detached.
Body: Over-under plain weave
Other: Evidence of structural padding on sole

Catalog no.: 42KA433 (FS68) 23904
Site: Benchmark Cave, Utah
Collector and date: UCRBASP, 1958
Cultural period: Pueblo II-Pueblo III
Construction technique: Plain weave
Dimensions: Length 24.5 cm, width 14.5 cm, depth
    2.26 cm
Active elements: Leaf element unspun, cortex intact
Average width: 0.55 cm
Passive elements: Leaf element unspun(?)
Number of passive units: 2
Number in unit: 1(?)
Average width: ?
Ties, loops, attachments: Heel: Loop of S-twisted leaf
    knotted to sole on one side then incorporated
    with an S-twisted leaf element and knotted, to
    form tie over foot
Shape: Left foot shaping, rounded toe and heel
Start: Warps are tied together in one knot at toe.
Body: Over-under plain weave using two layers(?) of
    wefts at a time, ending on sole for padding.
    Additional fibrous padding added to top of
    sandal, secured by side lacing. Knot visible on
    edge of sole
Finish: Knotted warps not visible on heel. Wefts
    appear to be folded over heel and tucked in
    sole.

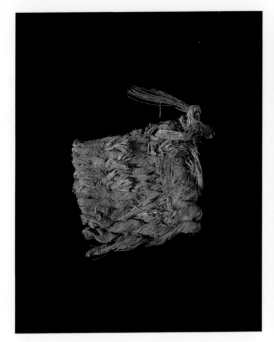

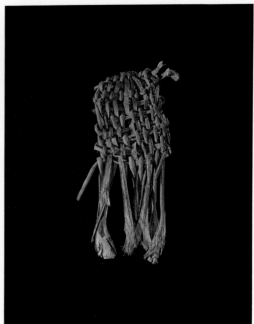

Catalog no.: 42KA433 (FS74.2) 23904
Site: Benchmark Cave, Utah
Collector and date: UCRBASP, 1958
Cultural period: Pueblo II-Pueblo III
Construction technique: Plain weave
Dimensions: Length 8.8 cm, width 8.9 cm, depth 1.2 cm
Active elements: Leaf element, some cortex intact, twisted S
Average width: 0.59 cm
Passive elements: Leaf element unspun, cortex intact
Number of passive units: 4
Number in unit: 1
Average width: 0.77 cm
Ties, loops, attachments: Edge: Shredded leaf element, tied and attached on corner of fragment with two knots
Shape: Fragmentary
Start and Finish: Missing
Body: Over-under plain weave for length of fragment
Other: Structural padding on sole. Added padding on top of sandal

Catalog no.: 42KA433 (FS77.5) 24133
Site: Benchmark Cave, Utah
Collector and date: UCRBASP, 1962
Cultural period: Pueblo II-Pueblo III
Construction technique: Plain weave
Dimensions: Length 14.7 cm, width 5.8 cm, depth 1.5 cm
Active elements: Leaf element unspun, cortex intact
Average width: 0.35 cm
Passive elements: Leaf element unspun, cortex intact
Number of passive units: 16
Number in unit: 1
Average width: 0.42 cm
Ties, loops, attachments: None apparent
Shape: Unfinished rectangular piece
Start: Eight warps are doubled to form 16 warps. Long weft piece is passed through the loop of the doubled warp, leaving a short end of weft at one side, which in turn is woven across the warp (plain weave), split at the end to pass over and under long weft.
Body: Long weft end is woven over-under with a splice on the third row.
Finish: Incomplete, warp ends left extended

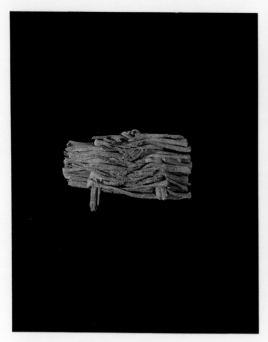 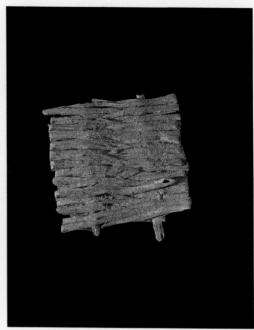

Catalog no.: 42KA433 (FS91.1) 24133
Site: Benchmark Cave, Utah
Collector and date: UCRBASP, 1962
Cultural period: Pueblo II-Pueblo III
Construction technique: Plain weave
Dimensions: Length 6.0 cm, width 10.5 cm, depth
   1.83 cm
Active elements: Leaf element unspun, cortex intact
Average width: 0.47 cm
Passive elements: Leaf element unspun, cortex intact
Number of passive units: 2
Number in unit: 1
Average width: 0.75 cm
Ties, loops, attachments: None apparent
Shape: Fragmentary
Start or Finish: Two knots at remaining end
Body: Over-under plain weave, long wefts encircle
   warps both tightly and loosely which extends the
   width of sandal beyond the warp edge.

Catalog no.: 42KA433 (FS91.2) 24133
Site: Benchmark Cave, Utah
Collector and date: UCRBASP, 1962
Cultural period: Pueblo II-Pueblo III
Construction technique: Plain weave
Dimensions: Length 12.0 cm, width 11.0 cm, depth
   0.35 cm
Active elements: Leaf element unspun, cortex intact
Average width: 0.57 cm
Passive elements: Leaf element unspun, cortex intact
Number of passive units: 2
Number in unit: 1
Average width: 0.64 cm
Ties, loops, attachments: None apparent
Shape: Fragmentary
Start and Finish: Missing
Body: Over-under plain weave. Wefts encircle
   warps both tightly and loosely which extends the
   width of sandal beyond the warp edge.
Other: Remnant of structural padding on sole

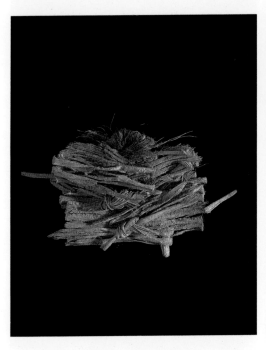

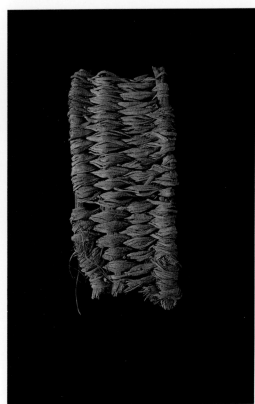

Catalog no.: 42KA433 (FS91.3) 24133
Site: Benchmark Cave, Utah
Collector and date: UCRBASP, 1962
Cultural period: Pueblo II-Pueblo III
Construction technique: Plain weave
Dimensions: Length 10 cm, width 11.5 cm, depth 0.82 cm
Active elements: Leaf element unspun, cortex intact
Average width: 0.55 cm
Passive elements: Leaf element unspun, cortex intact
Number of passive units: 2
Number in unit: 1(?)
Average width: 0.63 cm
Ties, loops, attachments: Two knotted wefts on surface, one attached
Shape: Fragmentary, heel or toe missing
Start or Finish: Warps are knotted on sole.
Body: Over-under plain weave. Wefts encircle warps both tightly and loosely which extends the width of sandal beyond the warp edge.
Other: Structural padding(?)

Catalog no.: 42KA433 (FS160.3) 23904
Site: Benchmark Cave, Utah
Collector and date: UCRBASP, 1962
Cultural period: Pueblo II-Pueblo III
Construction technique: Plain weave
Dimensions: Length 19.7 cm, width 8.6 cm, depth 1.0 cm
Active elements: Separated leaf element, unspun, cortex intact
Average width: 0.55 cm
Passive elements: Leaf element unspun, cortex intact
Number of passive units: 4
Number in unit: 1
Average width: 0.71 cm
Ties, loops, attachments: None apparent
Shape: Toe and heel missing
Start and Finish: Missing
Body: Over-under plain weave for length of sandal. Exhausted ends left frayed on sole
Other: Structural padding on sole

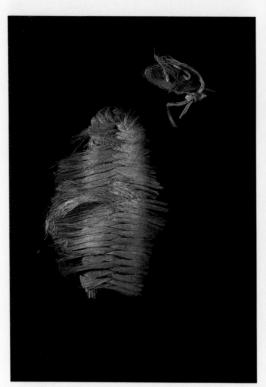

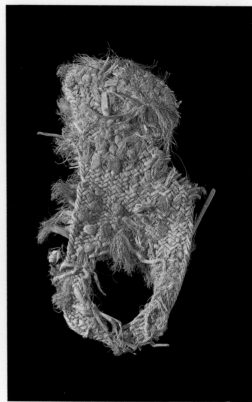

Catalog no.: 42SA736 (FS9.9) 24080
Site: Bernheimer Alcove, Utah
Collector and date: UCRBASP, 1961
Cultural period: Pueblo II
Construction technique: Plain weave
Dimensions: Length 15.50 cm, width 10.0 cm, depth 0.9 cm
Active elements: Leaf element unspun, cortex intact
Average width: 0.79 cm
Passive elements: Leaf element unspun, cortex intact
Number of passive units: 2
Number in unit: 2
Average width: 0.85 cm
Ties, loops, attachments: Leaf element ties are slightly entangled near sandal toe. Two knots are present.
Shape: Rounded toe, heel missing
Start: Warps are tied together in one knot at toe.
Body: Over-under plain weave beginning with narrow end of leaf element on top and ending with shredded wide ends on sole for padding. Wefts encircle warps both tightly and loosely extending width of sandal beyond warp edge.
Finish: Missing
Other: Structural padding on sole, charred

Catalog no.: 42SA736 (FS80.11) 24080
Site: Bernheimer Alcove, Utah
Collector and date: UCRBASP, 1961
Cultural period: Basketmaker III-Pueblo III
Construction technique: Plaited
Dimensions: Length 23.0 cm, width 9.7 cm, depth 1.5 cm
Active elements: Leaf element unspun, cortex intact
Average width: 0.32 cm
Passive elements: N/A
Ties, loops, attachments: Square knot on reverse edge
Shape: Right foot shaping, rounded toe and heel
Start: Active elements folded at toe
Body: 2/2 twill plaiting. Shifts are not visible due to heavy stitching and fraying. Exhausted ends left frayed on sole
Finish: It appears elements are looped around adjacent element. Heel area missing
Other: Stitching throughout sandal appears structural. Ends are left protruding on sole. Structural padding on sole

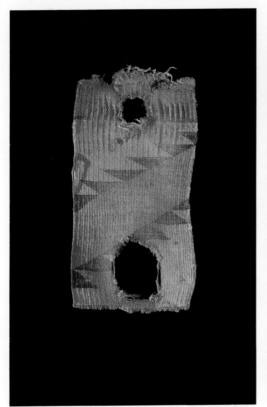
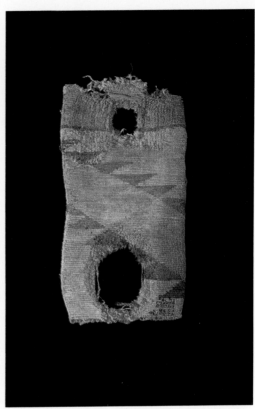

Catalog no.: 42SA736 (FS38.7) 24080
Site: Bernheimer Alcove, Utah
Collector and date: UCRBASP, 1961
Cultural period: Basketmaker II(?)
Construction technique: Composite
Dimensions: Length 21.0 cm, width 11.0 cm, depth
    0.42 cm
Active elements: Cordage, 2 ply, s-Z twist
Average width: 0.09 cm
Passive elements: Cordage, 2 ply, s-Z twist
Number of passive units: 47
Number in unit: 1 (except where doubled at toe)
Average width: 0.14 cm
Ties, loops, attachments: Toe: Stitched attachment at
    toe appears to be hide.
Shape: Left(?) foot shaping, squared toe and heel
Start: Warps appear woven singly near toe in 2/2
    twining then folded over a stick or rigid element
    and secured at two points. 2/2 twining continues
    over doubled warps. When secured, doubled
    warps are truncated.
Body: Triangular designs in natural dyed black,
    yellow, and green. Design same on both surfaces.
    Achieved with two wefts, one in natural which is
    static and carried selvage to selvage, while the
    dyed weft wraps around the warp and static
    weft. Dyed wefts weave back and forth in their
    own areas. The static weft gives a firm
    background and avoids slits or spaces between
    different weft colors. Five rows of 1/1 plain
    weave complete weaving at heel.
Finish: At heel warp ends are braided.

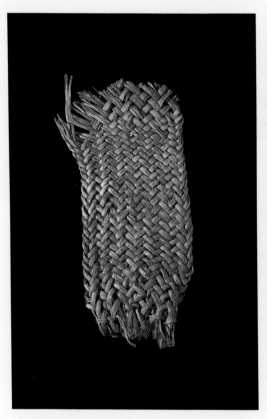
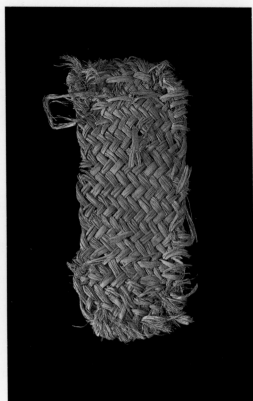

Catalog no.: 941

Site: Betatakin, Arizona

Collector and date: Byron Cummings, University of Utah Expedition, 1909

Cultural period: Pueblo III

Construction technique: Plaited

Dimensions: Length 20.0 cm, width 9.5 cm, depth 0.41 cm

Active elements: Leaf element unspun, cortex intact

Average width: 0.47 cm

Passive elements: N/A

Ties, loops, attachments: None apparent

Shape: Toe missing, straight heel with ends left exposed

Start: Missing

Body: 2/2 twill plaiting for length of sandal pulling in toward heel

Finish: At heel elements are twined from each edge toward center where twining is tied in a knot.

Catalog no.: 943

Site: Betatakin, Arizona

Collector and date: Byron Cummings, University of Utah Expedition, 1909

Cultural period: Pueblo III

Construction technique: Plaited

Dimensions: Length 23.30 cm, width 9.38 cm, depth 0.69 cm

Active elements: Leaf element unspun, cortex intact

Average width: 0.60 cm

Passive elements: N/A

Ties, loops, attachments: Edge: Loop remnants appear to be cordage 2 ply, z-S twist.

Shape: Right foot shaping, squared toe and rounded heel

Start: Active elements folded at toe

Body: 2/2 twill plaiting for length of sandal with a 2/3/2 shift at selvage

Finish: Horizontal leaf element added across heel. Active elements wrap around this bar and are clipped short on sole.

Other: Horizontal stitches of 4 rows across heel and 3 rows across toe appear structural. They are secured by encircling edge of sandal several times.

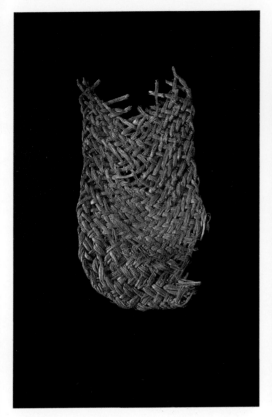

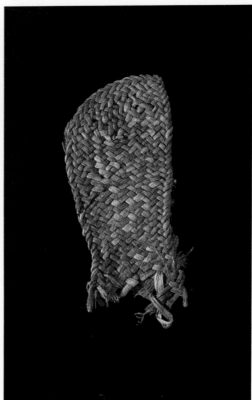

Catalog no.: 944
Site: Betatakin, Arizona
Collector and date: Byron Cummings, University of
  Utah Expedition, 1909
Cultural period: Pueblo III
Construction technique: Plaited
Dimensions: Length 19.0 cm, width 10.2 cm, depth
  0.6 cm
Active elements: Leaf element unspun, cortex intact
Average width: 0.45 cm
Passive elements: N/A
Ties, loops, attachments: None apparent
Shape: Rounded or tapered toe, heel missing
Start: Doubled elements are folded at toe with
  short ends overlapping.
Body: 2/2 twill plaiting over doubled elements for
  4.0 cm at which point doubled elements end and
  plaiting continues on single elements. Shift of 1/1
  at toe edge
Finish: Missing

Catalog no.: 945
Site: Betatakin, Arizona
Collector and date: Byron Cummings, University of
  Utah Expedition, 1909
Cultural period: Pueblo III
Construction technique: Plaited
Dimensions: Length 18.5 cm, width 9.0 cm, depth
  0.4 cm
Active elements: Leaf element unspun, cortex intact
Average width: 0.44 cm
Passive elements: N/A
Ties, loops, attachments: Toe: Two possible awl(?)
  holes Heel: Knotted remnant emerges on sole.
Shape: Left foot shaping, tapered toe, heel missing
Start: Active elements folded at toe
Body: 2/2 twill plaiting with shifts of 2/1/2 in toe
  area. Where sandal narrows five ends are turned
  180° and ended.
Finish: Missing

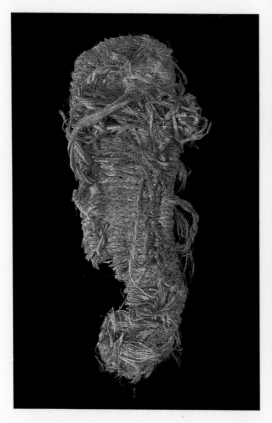 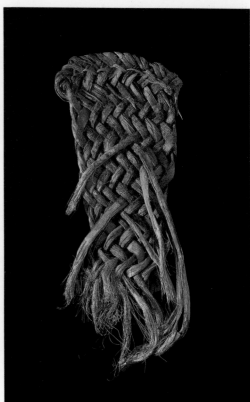

Catalog no.: 1273
Site: Betatakin, Arizona
Collector and date: Byron Cummings, University of
Utah Expedition, 1909
Cultural period: Pueblo III
Construction technique: Plain weave
Dimensions: Length 28.5 cm, width 10 cm, depth 1
cm
Active elements: Separated leaf elements, cortex
intact twisted S and Z
Average width: 0.4 cm
Passive elements: Three strand braid of leaf
elements, cortex intact
Number of passive units: 4
Number in unit: 1
Average width: 0.66 cm
Ties, loops, attachments: Toe: Leaf element on right
side and 2 ply z-S twist cordage on left. Heel:
Leaf element and knot remnants. Edge: Leaf
elements and 2 ply z-S twist cordage loop and
stitch through sandal up right side. At least 6
elements knot on sole of sandal. On left side at
instep several flat leaf elements stitch up side
with one long loop.
Shape: Slight left foot shaping, squared toe and
rounded heel
Start: Two braided leaf element warps folded at toe
(one inside the other) to form four warps
Body: Tightly packed plain weave continues to heel.
Weft appears gathered and twisted as it is
woven. From heel Z twist for 5.0 cm; S twist-3.0
cm; Z twist-4.5 cm, S twist-7 rows; Z twist-7
rows; S twist-5 rows; Z twist-1 row; S twist-1
row; Z twist-5 rows; S twist to toe

Finish: At heel warps appear knotted and tucked
back into sandal.

Catalog no.: 1271
Site: Betatakin, Arizona
Collector and date: Byron Cummings, University of
Utah Expedition, 1909
Cultural period: Pueblo III
Construction technique: Plaited
Dimensions: Length 19.0 cm, width 10.0 cm, depth
0.70 cm
Active elements: Leaf element, unspun, cortex intact
Average width: 0.88 cm
Passive elements: N/A
Ties, loops, attachments: None apparent
Shape: Slightly rounded toe. Sandal appears never
completed as elements eliminated for shaping
have been left untrimmed.
Start: Sixteen leaf elements with narrow ends at
toe have been twined with decorticated
untwisted fibers for one row of Z twining. The
16 narrow ends fold over twining and tip is
aligned with tips of 16 new ends forming a
splice. 2/2 plaiting begins incorporating spliced
elements with twining row appearing on one
side only.
Body: 2/2 plaiting continues until shaping requires
dropping active elements. Plaiting shifts in three
locations to 2/1/2 and drops a total of 6
elements for shaping.
Finish: At heel 8 elements are left unwoven on sole.
The remaining elements are doubled over a
transverse element and left protruding on upper
surface.

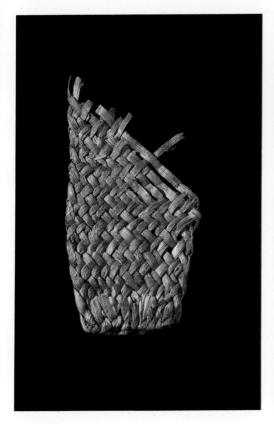

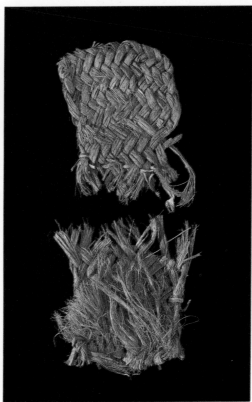

Catalog no.: 2800
Site: Betatakin, Arizona
Collector and date: Byron Cummings, University of
    Utah Expedition, 1909
Cultural period: Pueblo III
Construction technique: Plaited
Dimensions: Length 20.50 cm, width 10.25 cm,
    depth 0.50 cm
Active elements: Leaf element unspun, cortex intact
Average width: 0.47 cm
Passive elements: N/A
Ties, loops, attachments: None apparent
Shape: Squared heel, toe missing
Start: Missing
Body: 2/2 twill plaiting for length of sandal. Two
    elements are dropped near heel for shaping.
Finish: At heel a 2 ply cord forms a double bar that
    is knotted at one end. Every other active
    element loops around top cord and protrudes
    on upper side of sandal. Remaining elements
    encircle bottom cord and protrude on sole.

Catalog no.: 2819 A and B
Site: Betatakin, Arizona
Collector and date: Byron Cummings, University of
    Utah Expedition, 1909
Cultural period: Pueblo III
Construction technique: Plaited
Dimensions: A: Length 12.0 cm, width 10.25 cm,
    depth 0.75 cm. B: Length 14.0 cm, width 10.0
    cm, depth 0.65 cm
Active elements: Leaf element unspun, cortex intact
Average width: 0.67 cm
Passive elements: N/A
Ties, loops, attachments: Heel: On both edges of
    heel small leaf element knots remain.
Shape: Squared heel (A), slightly rounded toe (B)
Start: (B) Active elements are aligned parallel and
    doubled with narrow ends overlapping for a
    short distance. After one row of twining
    elements fold.
Body: 2/2 twill plaiting for length of sandals with
    doubled elements plaited at toe only. At
    midsection another row of twining is evident.
    Shift at selvage edge of 2/3/2.
Finish: At heel (B) half of the active elements are
    folded over a transverse bar with the remaining
    ends clipped short on sole. Weft ends on
    surface side kept long
Other: Sandal has broken into two sections.

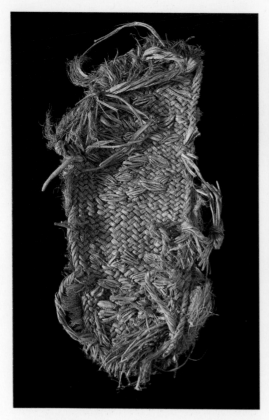

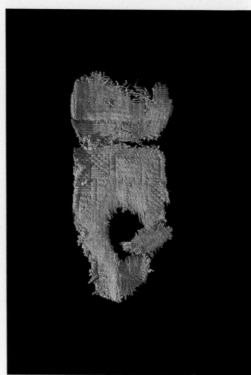

Catalog no.: 2846
Site: Betatakin, Arizona
Collector and date: Byron Cummings, University of
    Utah Expedition, 1909
Cultural period: Basketmaker III
Construction technique: Composite
Dimensions: Length 19.50 cm, width 8.50 cm, depth
    0.30 cm
Active elements: Cordage, 2 ply, z-S twist
Average width: 0.09 cm
Passive elements: Cordage, 3 ply, z-S twist
Number of passive units: 30
Number in unit: 1 (except where doubled at toe)
Average width: 0.15 cm
Ties, loops, attachments: None apparent
Shape: Not determinable, but other sandals of this
    type are scalloped toe and puckered heel.
Start: Probable scalloped toe start
Body: 2/2 alternate pair twining over doubled warps
    for forward one-third section of sandal at which
    point doubled warps end. Midsection appears to
    be twining and warp wrapping. Remaining length
    of sandal to heel woven in raised geometric
    pattern
Finish: Missing

58 Catalog no.: 2841
    Site: Betatakin, Arizona
    Collector and date: Byron Cummings, University of
        Utah Expedition, 1909
    Cultural period: Pueblo III
    Construction technique: Plaited
    Dimensions: Length 27.0 cm, width 11.0 cm, depth
        0.81 cm
    Active elements: Leaf element unspun, cortex intact
    Average width: 0.34 cm
    Passive elements: N/A
    Ties, loops, attachments: Toe: Loop of leaf element,
        twisted S. Edge: Loops and ties of leaf element
        twisted S.
    Shape: Left foot shaping, tapered toe and rounded
        heel.
    Start: Active elements folded at toe.
    Body: 2/2 twill plaiting for length of sandal.
        Exhausted ends left frayed on sole. Shifts at
        selvage of 2/3/2.
    Finish: Ends folded back into sandal.
    Other: Stitches of leaf element appear structural
        across heel and toe areas. Structural padding on
        sole

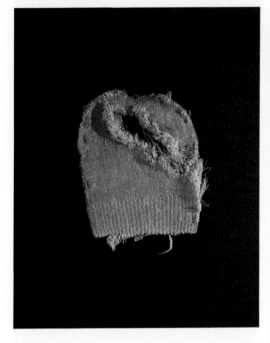
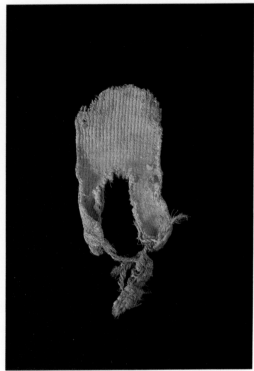

Catalog no.: 2847
Site: Betatakin, Arizona
Collector and date: Byron Cummings, University of
    Utah Expedition, 1909
Cultural period: Basketmaker III
Construction technique: Composite
Dimensions: Length 11.5 cm, width 9.50 cm
Active elements: Cordage, 2 ply, z-S twist
Average width: 0.11 cm
Passive elements: Cordage, 3 ply, z-S twist
Number of passive units: 29
Number in unit: 1 (except where doubled at toe)
Average width: 0.16 cm
Ties, loops, attachments: Edge: Remnant toe ties
Shape: Scalloped toe, heel missing
Start: Scalloped toe start
Body: 2/2 alternate pair twining over doubled warps
    for forward one-third section of sandal at which
    point doubled warps end. Remaining length of
    sandal to heel woven in raised geometric pattern
Finish: Missing
Other: Running stitches on left side of toe

Catalog no.: 2848
Site: Betatakin, Arizona
Collector and date: Byron Cummings, University of
    Utah Expedition, 1909
Cultural period: Basketmaker III
Construction technique: Composite
Dimensions: Length 15.0 cm, width 7.50 cm, depth
    0.362 cm
Active elements: Cordage, 2 ply, z-S twist
Average width: 0.09 cm
Passive elements: Cordage, 3 ply, z-S twist
Number of passive units: 25
Number in unit: 1
Average width: 0.16 cm
Ties, loops, attachments: Heel: Cordage, 2 ply S twist
    (each ply 2 ply, z-S twist). Cords from both sides
    of heel twisted and knotted. Edge: Possible awl(?)
    hole on left side
Shape: Unknown, fragmentary
Start: Missing
Body: Sole is worn, but a ridge appears every few
    rows indicating a possible row of 3 element
    twining, or possibly soumac. Heel has faint
    indication of knots which could be remnants of a
    raised geometric pattern.
Finish: Fragmentary, but there appears to be some
    wrapping at right edge. Heel cord is knotted.

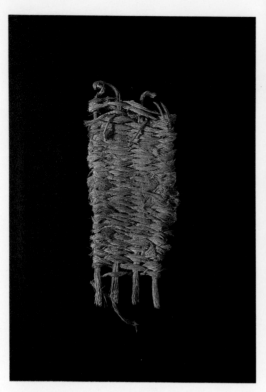

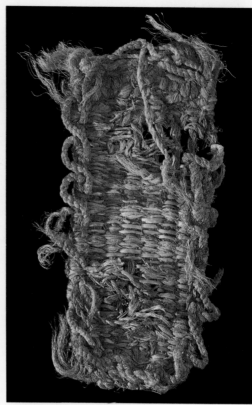

60   *Catalog no.:* 2849
      Site: Betatakin, Arizona
      Collector and date: Byron Cummings, University of
         Utah Expedition, 1909
      Cultural period: Pueblo III
      Construction technique: Plain weave
      Dimensions: Length 21.0 cm, width 7.0 cm, depth
         0.98 cm
      Active elements: Leaf element unspun, cortex intact
      Average width: 0.40 cm
      Passive elements: Leaf element unspun, cortex intact
      Number of passive units: 4
      Number in unit: 1
      Average width: 0.40 cm
      Ties, loops, attachments: Toe: Narrow leaf element
         encircles two middle warps. Edge: Knot on right
         edge
      Shape: Toe and heel missing
      Start: Missing, but position of warps indicates
         possibly tied in two groups
      Body: Over-under plain weave for length of sandal
      Finish: Missing

Catalog no.: 4935
Site: Bluff, Utah
Collector and date: Frank Hyde Collection, 1906-
   1920
Cultural period: Unknown
Construction technique: Plain weave
Dimensions: Length 28.0 cm, width 12.5 cm, depth
   1.18 cm
Active elements: Two types of elements: (A)
   Shredded leaf element slightly twisted S and Z
   and (B) a flat leaf element. Both with cortex
   intact
Average width: (A) 0.48 cm (B) 0.35 cm
Passive elements: Cordage, 2 ply, s-Z twist
Number of passive units: 8
Number in unit: 1
Average width: 0.78 cm
Ties, loops, attachments: Cordage, 2 ply, s-Z twist is
   looped around entire perimeter of sandal in
   overlapping technique. Majority of loops are
   attached by knotting.
Material: Yucca sp., animal hair
Shape: Squared toe and heel
Start: Warps appear aligned parallel with ends left
   protruding at toe.
Body: Over-under plain weave for length of sandal.
   Horizontal striping occurs by using two types of
   wefts, one a twisted leaf element and the other
   a flat leaf element. At both selvages, and at toe
   and heel ends, a supplementary two-ply strand is
   stitched lengthwise over the woven surface. Ends
   are frayed on sole.
Finish: At heel warps appear tucked back into body
   of sandal.
Other: Stitches and padding structural

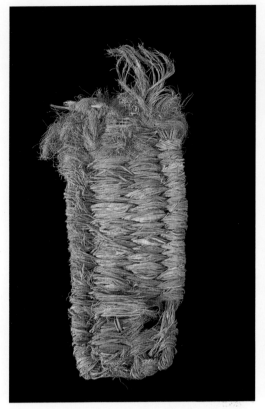
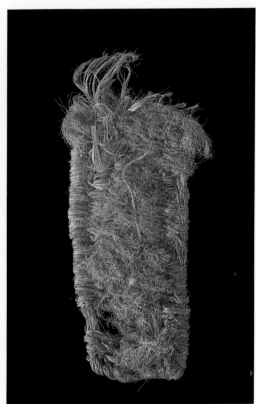

Catalog no.: 42SA356 (FS9.2) 24170
Site: Castle Wash Sites, Utah
Collector and date: Test Site, UCRBASP, 1962
Cultural period: Pueblo II
Construction technique: Plain weave
Dimensions: Length 23.0 cm, width 10.0 cm, depth
   1.28 cm
Active elements: Shredded leaf element unspun,
   cortex intact
Average width: 0.70 cm
Passive elements: Shredded leaf element 2 ply, lightly
   spun z, twisted S, cortex intact
Number of passive units: 4
Number in unit: 1
Average width: 0.92 cm
Ties, loops, attachments: Toe: Remnant of cordage
   tie 2 ply, z-S twist, knotted to a piece of leaf
   element on left side of toe
Shape: Right(?) foot shaping, squared toe and
   rounded heel
Start: At toe a 2 ply z-S twist cordage is knotted at
   one end and appears woven or twined around
   warps, with several areas evident of a portion of
   warp, or vertical element, wrapping around this
   cordage. This anchors the wefts which are
   frayed and fringed at toe.
Body: Over-under plain weave for length of sandal
   with exhausted ends left frayed on sole
Finish: At heel warps appear looped around
   adjacent warps. Some at heel are missing.
Other: Structural padding on sole

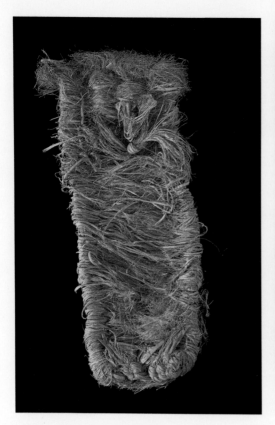 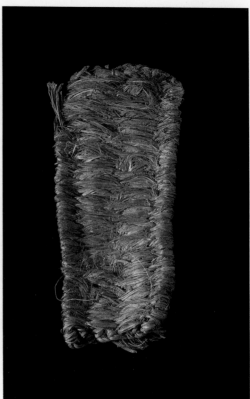

62   *Catalog no.:* 42SA356 (FS19.1) 24170
     Site: Castle Wash Sites, Utah
     Collector and date: Test Site, UCRBASP, 1962
     Cultural period: Pueblo II-Pueblo II
     Construction technique: Plain weave
     Dimensions: Length 28.0 cm, width 11.0 cm, depth 1.27 cm
     Active elements: Separated leaf element unspun, cortex intact
     Average width: 0.7 cm
     Passive elements: Separated leaf elements 2 ply, z-S twist, cortex intact
     Number of passive units: 4
     Number in unit: 1
     Average width: 1.0 cm
     Ties, loops, attachments: Toe: Loop tie passes under the body of the sandal between the 1st and 2nd warps and 2nd and 4th warps; ends tied on top to form loop.
     Shape: Right foot shaping, squared toe and rounded heel
     Start or Finish: First weft row is woven in about 2 cm from the end. It is anchored to the warp by ties across the width of the sandal with at least one of the wraps going through the warps as well as around the weft. A short length of 2 ply z-S twist cordage is visible and appears to be part of anchoring system for wefts. The ends are frayed.
     Body: Over-under plain weave, most elements ending on sole for padding
     Finish: Warp ends at heel are successively looped around and under adjacent warps from right to left side. Captured ends are clipped on top.
     Other: Structural padding on sole

Catalog no.: 1113
Site: Cave near Navajo Mountain, Utah
Collector and date: Byron Cummings, University of Utah Expedition, 1912
Cultural period: Unknown
Construction technique: Plain weave
Dimensions: Length 22.5 cm, width 9.5 cm, depth 1.0 cm
Active elements: Leaf element unspun, cortex intact
Average width: 0.71 cm
Passive elements: Separated leaf elements, cortex intact, 2 ply, spun slighty z-S twist
Number of passive units: 4
Number in unit: 1
Average width: 0.87 cm
Ties, loops, attachments: None apparent
Shape: Squared toe and heel
Start: Four warps are untwisted at toe to make 8 elements which are secured with 2 rows of twining.
Body: 1/1 plain weave continues from twined toe to heel.
Finish: At heel the two elements comprising each warp are used separately, wrapped around adjacent warp and tucked back into sandal.
Other: Structural padding on sole

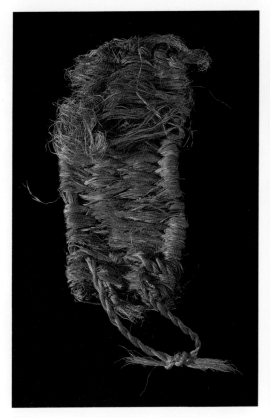
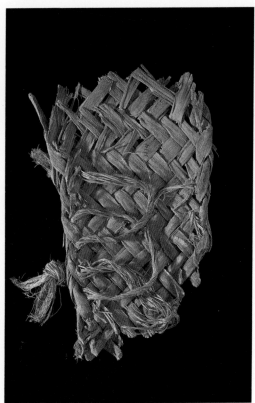

Catalog no.: 1112
Site: Cave near Navajo Mountain, Utah
Collector and date: Byron Cummings, University of
Utah Expedition, 1912
Cultural period: Unknown
Construction technique: Plain weave
Dimensions: Length 23.5 cm, width 10.4 cm, depth
1.4 cm
Active elements: Leaf element unspun, cortex intact
Average width: 0.78 cm
Passive elements: Separated leaf elements, cortex
intact, 2 ply, z-S twist
Number of passive units: 4
Number in unit: 1
Average width: 0.64 cm
Ties, loops, attachments: Heel: Two lengths of
cordage, 2 ply, s-Z twist are wrapped around
either side of warp; two ends are knotted
together on the sole, and the remaining two
ends form a heel loop that is knotted together.
Shape: Left foot shaping, squared toe and heel
Start: Four warps untwisted at toe to make eight
elements, which are secured with 2 rows of
twining
Body: 1/1 plain weave continues from twined toe to
heel.
Finish: At heel the two elements comprising each
warp are used separately, wrapped around and
secured to adjacent warp and tucked back into
sandal.
Other: Structural padding on sole

Catalog no.: 1114
Site: Cave near Navajo Mountain, Utah
Collector and date: Byron Cummings, University of
Utah Expedition, 1912
Cultural period: Unknown
Construction technique: Plaited
Dimensions: Length 24.0 cm, width 13.50 cm, depth
1.10 cm
Active elements: 1.28 cm
Passive elements: N/A
Ties, loops, attachments: Edge: Remaining on one
edge only are loops of leaf element twisted Z.
Loops anchored on sole with overhand knots
and worked back into sandal with a backstitch.
New elements are added by knotting.
Shape: Toe and heel missing, fragmentary
Start: Missing
Body: 2/2 plaiting for length of fragment
Finish: Missing

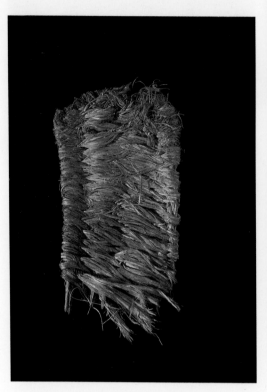

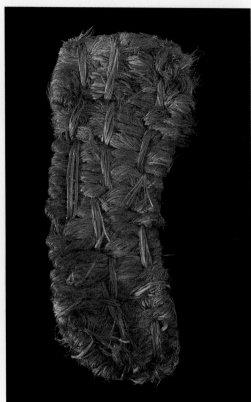

64   *Catalog no.:* 1115
Site: Cave near Navajo Mountain, Utah
Collector and date: Byron Cummings, University of
   Utah Expedition, 1912
Cultural period: Unknown
Construction technique: Plain weave
Dimensions: Length 18.0 cm, width 10.0 cm, depth
   1.0 cm
Active elements: Leaf element unspun, cortex intact
Average width: 0.63 cm
Passive elements: Separated leaf elements, cortex
   intact, 2 ply z-S twist
Number of passive units: 4
Number in unit: 1
Average width: 0.78 cm
Ties, loops, attachments: None apparent
Shape: Squared toe, heel missing
Start: Four warps are untwisted at toe to make 8
   elements, which are secured with 2 rows of
   twining.
Body: 1/1 plain weave continues from twined toe to
   heel.
Finish: Missing
Other: Structural padding on sole

Catalog no.: 1116
Site: Cave near Navajo Mountain, Utah
Collector and date: Byron Cummings, University of
   Utah Expedition, 1912
Cultural period: Unknown
Construction technique: Plain weave
Dimensions: Length 28.5 cm, width 12.0 cm, depth
   2.03 cm
Active elements: Leaf element unspun, cortex intact;
   loosely twisted, mostly z
Average width: 1.09 cm
Passive elements: Separated leaf elements, cortex
   intact, slightly spun Z and twisted S
Number of passive units: 4
Number in unit: 1
Average width: 0.61 cm
Ties, loops, attachments: None apparent
Shape: Left foot shaping, squared toe and rounded
   heel
Start: Warps appear knotted at toe in two groups
   of 2 warps each.
Body: 1/1 plain weave from toe to heel. Three
   reinforcing rows from toe to heel and back in
   stitches of separated leaf elements, cortex intact,
   unspun and knotted on sole
Finish: At heel warps are separated and wrapped
   around adjacent warp, pulled fairly tight and
   tucked back into sandal forming a rounded heel.
Other: Structural padding on sole

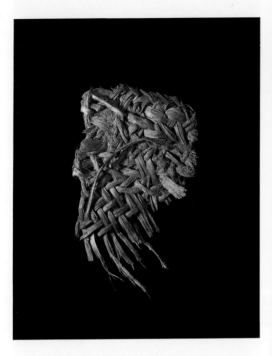

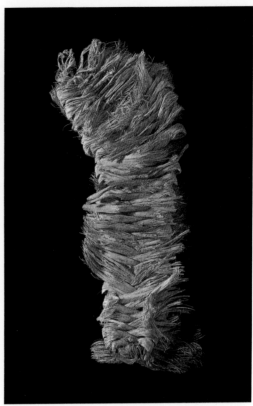

Catalog no.: 1117
Site: Cave near Navajo Mountain, Utah
Collector and date: Byron Cummings, University of
 Utah Expedition, 1912
Cultural period: Unknown
Construction technique: Plaited
Dimensions: Length 18.0 cm, width 9.50 cm, depth
 0.32 cm
Active elements: Leaf element unspun, cortex intact
Passive elements: N/A
Ties, loops, attachments: None apparent
Shape: Squared toe, fragmentary
Start: Six-eight elements doubled at toe to form
 12-16 elements
Body: 2/2 plaiting for toe area and rear portion.
 Forward section includes approximately 9
 transverse elements obliterating exact
 interlacement in this area.
Finish: Missing

Catalog no.: 42SA678 (FS9.2) 24068
Site: Coptor Ledge, Utah
Collector and date: UCRBASP 1961
Cultural period: Pueblo II
Construction technique: Plain weave
Dimensions: Length 26.0 cm, width 9.50 cm, depth
 2.50 cm
Active elements: Leaf element unspun, cortex intact
Average width: 0.7 cm
Passive elements: Leaf element unspun, cortex intact
Number of passive units: 2
Number in unit: 1
Average width: 0.6 cm
Ties, loops, attachments: None apparent
Shape: Rounded toe and heel
Start: Toe start fragmented
Body: Over-under plain weave beginning with
 narrow ends of leaf element on top and ending
 with shredded wide ends on sole for padding.
 Ends extend beyond body of sandal.
Finish: One knot of warp ends, structure of other
 fragmented ends uncertain
Other: Structural padding on sole

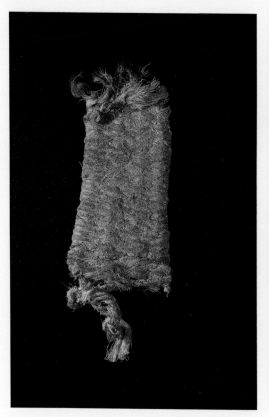
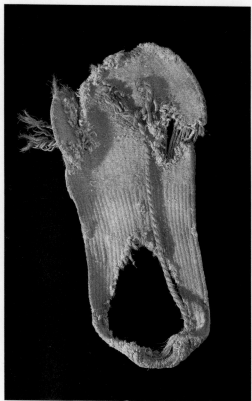

66 Catalog no.: 7167
Site: Cottonwood Wash, Utah
Collector and date: Ben and Hyrum Perkins, Hans
    Bayles, Platte Lyman, and Kuman Jones in 1892
    for the World's Fair in Chicago
Cultural period: Unknown
Construction technique: Plain weave
Dimensions: Length 23.0 cm, width 9.0 cm, depth
    1.0 cm
Active elements: Shredded leaf element,
    decorticated, twisted S and Z
Average width: 0.37 cm
Passive elements: Cordage, 2 ply s-Z twist
Number of passive units: 4
Number in unit: 1
Average width: 0.39 cm
Ties, loops, attachments: Toe: 2 ply, z-S twist cordage
    looped through center of warp fold. Edge: A
    short length of 2 ply, z-S twist cordage pierces
    edge of sandal with both ends emerging on
    upper surface.
Shape: Probable rounded toe, although
    disarticulating, heel missing
Start: Center warp folds creating two warps. Two
    outside warps are loose with shredding ends.
Body: Tightly packed plain weave for length of
    sandal. Shredded yucca weft appears gathered
    together for appropriate width of weft and
    twisted as it is woven. This gives an "S" twist in
    one direction and a "Z" twist in the opposite
    direction.
Finish: Missing
Other: Charring on heel warp ends

Catalog no.: 7169
Site: Cottonwood Wash, Utah
Collector and date: Ben and Hyrum Perkins, Hans
    Bayles, Platte Lyman, and Kuman Jones in 1892
    for Utah exhibition at Chicago World's Fair
Cultural period: Basketmaker III
Construction technique: Composite
Dimensions: Length 24.4 cm, width 14.0 cm, depth
    0.80 cm
Active elements: Cordage, 2 ply, z-S twist
Average width: 0.09 cm
Passive elements: Cordage, 3 ply, z-S twist
Number of passive units: 30
Number in unit: 1 (except where doubled at toe)
Average width: 0.25 cm
Ties, loops, attachments: Toe: Cordage, loop at toe 2
    ply, z-S twist. Heel: A length of cordage, 2 ply z-s
    twist, is knotted at right side of sandal and
    extends to toe loop.
Shape: Left(?) foot shaping, scalloped toe, puckered
    heel
Start: Scalloped toe start
Body: 2/2 alternate pair twining over doubled warps
    for forward one-third section of sandal at which
    point doubled warps end. Remaining length of
    sandal to heel woven in raised geometric pattern
Finish: Puckered heel finish. Heel cords missing

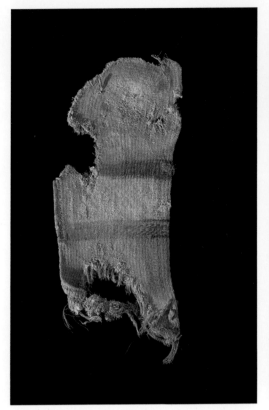
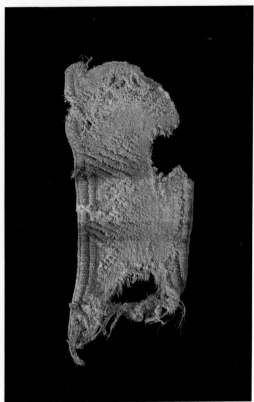

Catalog no.: 7172

Site: Cottonwood Wash, Utah

Collector and date: Ben and Hyrum Perkins, Hans Bayles, Platte Lyman, and Kuman Jones in 1892 for Utah exhibition at Chicago World's Fair

Cultural period: Basketmaker III (?)

Construction technique: Composite

Dimensions: Length 23.5 cm, width 9.90 cm, depth 0.46 cm

Active elements: Cordage, 2 ply, z-S twist

Average width: 0.15 cm

Passive elements: Cordage, 3 ply, z-S twist

Number of passive units: 36

Number in unit: 1

Average width: 0.12 cm

Ties, loops, attachments: Toe: Leaf tie remnant stitched on sole. Hide element protrudes near left side of toe. Heel: Cordage, tie remnant 3 ply, s-Z twist. Hide element protrudes on right side of heel. Edges: Knot remnants protrude on sole.

Shape: Left foot shaping, rounded toe and possible puckered heel

Start: Eighteen cords are looped at toe to form 36 warps. Twining begins at toe.

Body: Raised geometric pattern design on sole appears to begin at toe. Two colored bands at midsection use dyed weft elements. One band has a black stripe with two narrow stripes of brown/black on both sides. The second band toward the heel consists of a central stripe in brown/black and natural in an irregular diagonal pattern. A narrow black stripe borders center area. Diagonal pattern does not appear on sole.

Finish: Possible Puckered heel finish

Other: Because bar shapes on sole are fairly large, the number of weft wraps for raised area may have been increased. Small piece of hide wraps around heel tie.

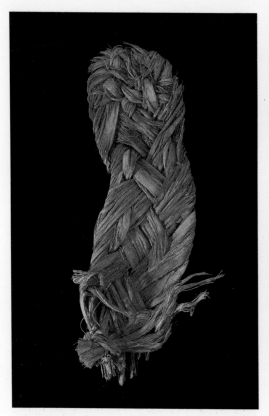

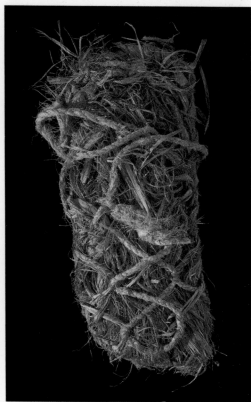

68   *Catalog no.:* 7173

Site: Cottonwood Wash, Utah

Collector and date: Ben and Hyrum Perkins, Hans Bayles, Platte Lyman, and Kuman Jones in 1892 for Utah exhibition at Chicago World's Fair.

Cultural period: Unknown

Construction technique: Plaited

Dimensions: Length 27.0 cm, width 8.0 cm, depth 0.82 cm

Active elements: Leaf element unspun, cortex intact

Average width: 0.48 cm

Passive elements: N/A

Ties, loops, attachments: Heel: Remnant of tie or loop leaf element around right side

Shape: Right foot shaping, rounded toe and heel

Start: Two leaf elements doubled at toe

Body: Four strand oblique plaiting for length of sandal (i.e., a four-strand braiding technique, from left under 1, from right over 1, under 1, etc.) Two smaller leaf elements are knotted at toe and stitched across toe, down both sides, and join with warp elements for finish.

Finish: At heel two active elements and stitching elements are bundled and wrapped with narrow leaf element and knotted.

Other: Shaping achieved by pulling tighter at instep

Catalog no.: 7176

Site: Cottonwood Wash, Utah

Collector and date: Ben and Hyrum Perkins, Hans Bayles, Platte Lyman, and Kuman Jones in 1892 for Utah exhibition at World's Fair in Chicago

Cultural period: Unknown

Construction technique: Plaited

Dimensions: Length 27.0 cm, width 12.0 cm, depth 1.50 cm (without padding)

Active elements: Leaf element, unspun, cortex intact

Average width: 0.71 cm

Passive elements: N/A

Ties, loops, attachments: Edge: Leaf elements are sewn in loops down each side, one 2 ply s-Z twist, cord laces through loops at toe to middle of sandal. Another 2 ply s-Z cord laces loops together at heel to mid section.

Shape: Rounded toe, straight heel with rounded corners

Start: Elements doubled at toe

Body: Exact interlacement interval not evident without removing padding. An additional running stitch appears on sole.

Finish: At heel ends appear folded over an additional leaf element and left protruding on sole.

Other: Yucca padding fills topside of sandal under laces with no wear indentations but sole of sandal is very worn.

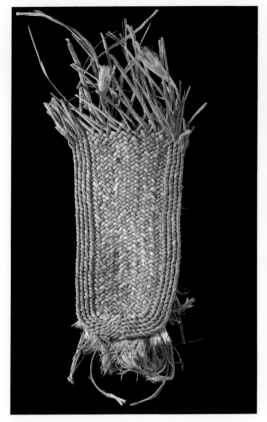 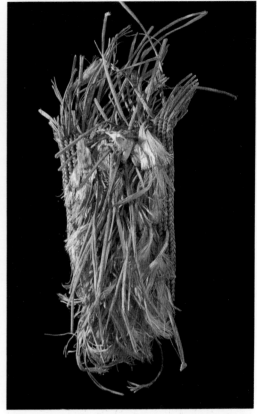

Catalog no.: 7175

Site: Cottonwood Wash, Utah

Collector and date: Ben and Hyrum Perkins, Hans
    Bayles, Platte Lyman, and Kuman Jones in 1892
    for Utah exhibition at Chicago World's Fair.

Cultural period: Unknown

Construction technique: Plaited

Dimensions: Length 18.5 cm, width 10.0 cm, depth
    0.62 cm

Active elements: Leaf element unspun, cortex intact

Average width: 0.30 cm

Passive elements: N/A

Ties, loops, attachments: None apparent

Shape: Rounded finished end

Start: Active elements fold from each side toward
    the center where they are plaited tightly to
    create four ridges.

Body: 2/2 twill plaiting for length of sandal with
    shifts of 2/1/2. Four ridges from start are carried
    down both sides.

Finish: Unknown

Other: Sandal appears never finished as elements
    are left unwoven and ends are untrimmed on
    sole.

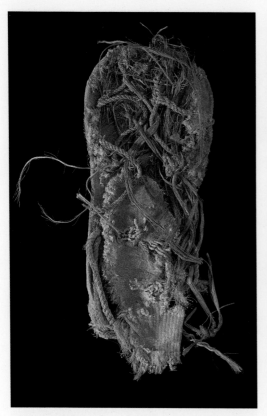
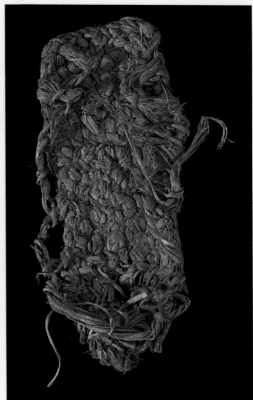

Catalog no.: 7177
Site: Cottonwood Wash, Utah
Collector and date: Ben and Hyrum Perkins, Hans
    Bayles, Platte Lyman, and Kuman Jones in 1892
    for Utah exhibition at Chicago World's Fair
Cultural period: Basketmaker III
Construction technique: Composite
Dimensions: Length 30.0 cm, width 12.5 cm, depth
    0.45 cm
Active elements: Cordage, 2 ply, z-S twist
Average width: 0.19 cm
Passive elements: Cordage, 3 ply, z-S twist
Number of passive units: 30
Number in unit: 1 (except where doubled at toe)
Average width: 0.12 cm
Ties, loops, attachments: Toe: Leaf element is
    knotted at toe then crisscrosses edge cordage.
    Edge: Cordage, 3 ply Z twist (each ply 2 ply z-S
    twist) begins at toe edges then loops and
    stitches along both sides to heel. Knot remnants
    protrude on sole.
Shape: Scalloped toe, rounded heel
Start: Scalloped toe start
Body: 2/2 alternate pair twining over doubled warps
    for forward one-third section of sandal at which
    point doubled warps end. Remaining length of
    sandal to heel woven in raised geometric pattern
Finish: Sandal mend forms heel.
Other: Patch on heel is a piece of composite sandal
    stitched to original sandal. Shredded yucca
    tucked into toe area

Catalog no.: 7178
Site: Cottonwood Wash, Utah
Collector and date: Ben and Hyrum Perkins, Hans
    Bayles, Platte Lyman, and Kuman Jones in 1892
    for Utah exhibition at Chicago World's Fair.
Cultural period: Unknown
Construction technique: Plaited
Dimensions: Length 30.0 cm, width 13.5 cm, depth
    1.0 cm
Active elements: Leaf element unspun, cortex intact
Average width: 0.45 cm
Passive elements: N/A
Ties, loops, attachments: Heel and Edge: Two leaf
    elements lightly twisted S together to form edge
    loops and heel loop
Shape: Left(?) foot shaping, rounded toe, gathered
    heel
Start: Active elements folded at toe
Body: 2/2 twill plaiting. Shifts not determinable due
    to stitching
Finish: Active elements gathered together at heel
    with a yucca strand
Other: Vertical and horizontal stitching

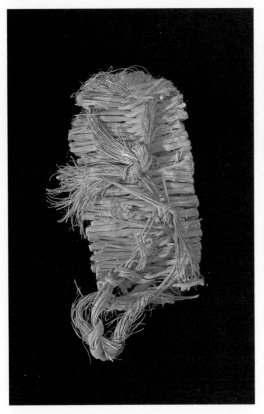
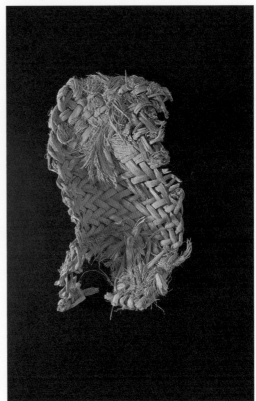

Catalog no.: 42KA241 (FS1) 23879
Site: Davis Kiva Site, Utah
Collector and date: UCRBASP, 1957
Cultural period: Pueblo II-Pueblo III
Construction technique: Plain weave
Dimensions: Length 18 cm, width 10 cm, depth 1.2
   cm
Active elements: Leaf element unspun, cortex intact
Average width: 0.57 cm
Passive elements: Leaf element unspun, cortex intact
Number of passive units: 2
Number in unit: 1
Average width: 0.79 cm
Ties, loops, attachments: Toe: Decorticated leaf
   element looped around sandal. Heel:
   Decorticated leaf element, S and Z twist,
   knotted at 3 places. Partially decorticated leaf
   element knotted to toe and heel loops
Shape: Rounded toe, heel missing
Start: Warps are tied together in one knot at toe,
   stitching around knot.
Body: Over-under plain weave beginning with
   narrow ends of leaf element on top and ending
   with shredded wide ends on sole for padding.
   Long wefts encircle warps tightly and loosely
   extending width of sandal beyond warp edges.
Finish: Missing
Other: Structural padding on sole

Catalog no.: 42KA241 (FS12) 23879
Site: Davis Kiva Site, Utah
Collector and date: UCRBASP, 1957
Cultural period: Pueblo II-Pueblo III
Construction technique: Plaited
Dimensions: Length 18.2 cm, width 9.3 cm, depth
   0.53 cm
Active elements: Leaf element unspun, cortex intact
Average width: 0.49 cm
Passive elements: N/A
Ties, loops, attachments: Edge: Two ties, one on each
   edge of shredded leaf element twisted Z. Both
   fold over plaiting at selvage.
Shape: Squared toe and heel
Start: Doubled active elements folded at toe
Body: 2/2 twill plaiting over doubled elements for
   one-third of sandal at which point doubled
   elements end and 2/2 plaiting continues using
   single elements for length of sandal.
Finish: Disarticulating, but it appears active elements
   wrap over a transverse bar at heel.

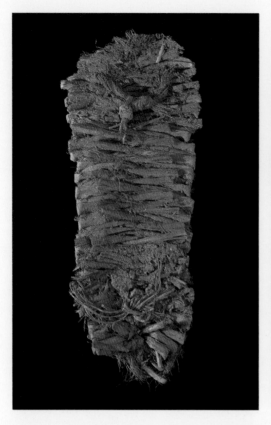
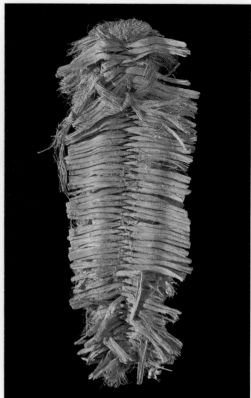

72 *Catalog no.:* 42KA241 (FS20) 23879
Site: Davis Kiva Site, Utah
Collector and date: UCRBASP, 1957
Cultural period: Pueblo II-Pueblo III
Construction technique: Plain weave
Dimensions: Length 26 cm, width 10.5 cm, depth 1.5
   cm
Active elements: Leaf element unspun, cortex intact
Average width: 0.67 cm
Passive elements: Leaf element unspun, cortex intact
Number of passive units: 2
Number in unit: 1
Average width: 1.0 cm
Ties, loops, attachments: Toe: Loop of leaf element,
   cortex partially gone, z twist, passed under sole
   and knotted on top. Remnant of tie knotted into
   loop. Heel: Loop partially attached and knotted
Shape: Left foot shaping, rounded toe and heel
Start: Two warps are tied together at toe in one
   knot.
Body: Over-under plain weave, beginning with
   narrow ends of leaf element on top near center,
   and ending with shredded wide ends on sole for
   padding
Finish: At heel, warps are knotted together.
Other: Structural padding on sole

Catalog no.: 42KA241 (FS21) 23879
Site: Davis Kiva Site, Utah
Collector and date: UCRBASP, 1957
Cultural period: Pueblo II-Pueblo III
Construction technique: Plain weave
Dimensions: Length 27.5 cm, width 10.5 cm, depth
   1.70 cm
Active elements: Leaf element unspun, cortex intact
Average width: 0.50 cm
Passive elements: Leaf element unspun, cortex intact
Number of passive units: 2
Number in unit: 1
Average width: 0.90 cm
Ties, loops, attachments: Toe: Tie of leaf element
   unspun, cortex partially gone; passed under sole
   and tied(?); remnant of lacing attached to toe
   loop by knot
Shape: Rounded toe and heel
Start: Warp elements are tied together in one knot
   at toe
Body: Over-under plain weave, beginning with
   narrow ends of leaf element on top and ending
   with shredded wide ends on sole for padding.
   Ends extend beyond body of sandal.
Finish: Warps knotted at heel
Other: Structural padding on sole

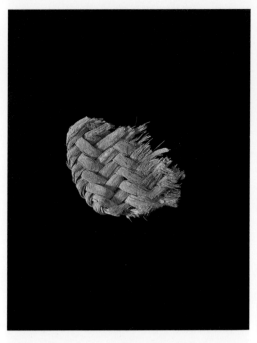

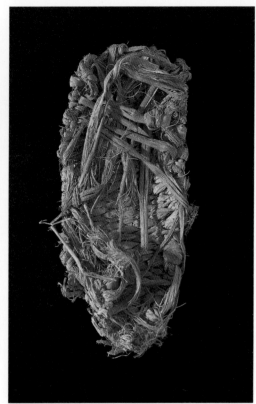

Catalog no.: 42KA241 (FS22) 23879
Site: Davis Kiva Site, Utah
Collector and date: UCRBASP, 1957
Cultural period: Pueblo II-Pueblo III
Construction technique: Plaited
Dimensions: Length 7.4 cm, width 7.52 cm, depth 0.58 cm
Active elements: Leaf element unspun, cortex intact
Average width: 0.81 cm
Passive elements: N/A
Ties, loops, attachments: None apparent
Shape: Rounded toe, fragmentary
Start: Active elements folded at toe
Body: 2/2 twill plaiting for length of fragment
Finish: Missing

Catalog no.: 42KA241 (FS33) 23879
Site: Davis Kiva, Utah
Collector and date: UCRBASP, 1957
Cultural period: Pueblo III
Construction technique: Twined
Dimensions: Length 22.8 cm, width 10.5 cm, depth 0.77 cm
Active elements: Leaf element unspun, cortex intact
Average width: 0.44 cm
Passive elements: Leaf element unspun, cortex intact
Number of passive units: 8
Number in unit: 1
Average width: 0.48 cm
Ties, loops, attachments: Toe: Leaf element ties. Heel: Leaf element ties, including two with wide ends extending on upper surface. Edge: Side loops of leaf element with some lacing across sandal still extant
Shape: Rounded toe and heel
Start: Eight warp leaf elements knotted (or wrapped) around first weft element and left protruding on upper surface
Body: 1/1 simple twining for length of sandal
Finish: At heel, broad ends of warp leaf elements protrude; twining appears to taper to tighten and narrow.

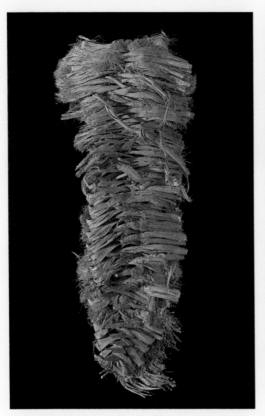 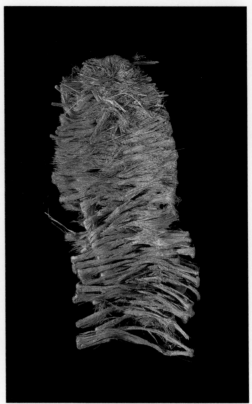

74   Catalog no.: 42KA241 AR041 23879
     Site: Davis Kiva Site, Utah
     Collector and date: UCRBASP, 1957
     Cultural period: Pueblo II-Pueblo III
     Construction technique: Plain weave
     Dimensions: Length 28.5 cm, width 12.5 cm, depth
        1.31 cm
     Active elements: Leaf element unspun, cortex intact
     Average width: 0.61 cm
     Passive elements: Leaf element unspun, cortex intact
     Number of passive units: 2
     Number in unit: 1
     Average width: 0.8 cm
     Ties, loops, attachments: Toe: Loop of leaf element
        unspun, cortex intact, passed under ball of foot
        and knotted on top
     Shape: Squared toe, gradually narrowing toward
        heel
     Start: Two warps are tied together in one knot at
        toe.
     Body: Over-under plain weave, beginning with
        narrow ends of leaf element on top and ending
        with shredded wide ends on sole for padding.
        Ends extend beyond body of sandal.
     Finish: Warps are tied together in a knot.
     Other: Structural padding on sole

Catalog no.: 42KA241 AR105 23879
Site: Davis Kiva Site, Utah
Collector and date: UCRBASP, 1957
Cultural period: Pueblo II-Pueblo III
Construction technique: Plain weave
Dimensions: Length 22.4 cm, width 9.8 cm, depth
   0.82 cm
Active elements: Leaf element unspun, cortex intact
Average width: 0.32 cm
Passive elements: Leaf element unspun, cortex intact
Number of passive units: 2
Number in unit: 1
Average width: 0.60 cm
Ties, loops, attachments: None apparent
Shape: Rounded toe, heel missing
Start: Two leaf warps tied together in one knot at
   toe
Body: Over-under plain weave, beginning with
   narrow end of leaf element on top and ending
   with shredded wide ends on sole for padding
Finish: Heel missing
Other: Structural padding on sole

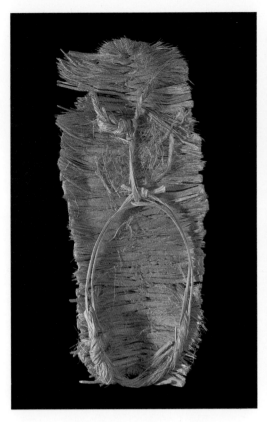
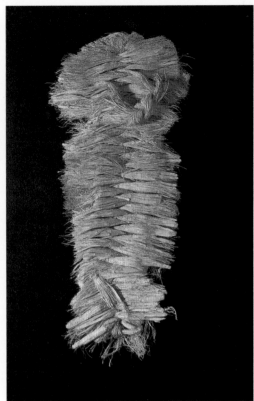

Catalog no.: 42KA241 AR4009 94.1 23879
Site: Davis Kiva Site, Utah
Collector and date: UCRBASP, 1958
Cultural period: Pueblo II-Pueblo III
Construction technique: Plain weave
Dimensions: Length 26.0 cm, width 11.0 cm, depth 1.05 cm
Active elements: Leaf element unspun, cortex intact
Average width: 0.30 cm
Passive elements: Leaf element unspun, cortex intact
Number of passive units: 2
Number in unit: 2
Average width: 0.65 cm
Ties, loops, attachments: Toe: Leaf element twisted S loops around toe area and knots. An instep loop attaches to toe loop and to large knotted loop that extends around heel.
Shape: Rounded toe and squared heel
Start: Warps are tied in one knot at toe. Stitching around knot
Body: Over-under plain weave, beginning with narrow ends of leaf element on top and ending with shredded wide ends on sole for padding. Wefts encircle warps both tightly and loosely which extends the width of sandal beyond the warp edge.
Finish: Warp ends tied in one knot at heel
Other: Structural padding on sole

Catalog no.: 42KA235 (FS10)
Site: Davis Pool Site, Utah
Collector and date: UCRBASP, 1957
Cultural period: Pueblo II-Pueblo III
Construction technique: Plain weave
Dimensions: Length 25.4 cm, width 12.5 cm, depth 1.80 cm
Active elements: Leaf element unspun, cortex intact
Average width: 0.63 cm
Passive elements: Leaf element unspun, cortex intact
Number of passive units: 2
Number in unit: 2
Average width: 1.14 cm
Ties, loops, attachments: Toe: Leaf element looped around warps at toe area and tied in a knot on surface
Shape: Rounded toe and squared heel
Start: Warps are tied together in one knot at toe. Stitching around knot
Body: Over-under plain weave, beginning with narrow ends of leaf element on top and ending with shredded wide ends on sole for padding. Wefts encircle warps both tightly and loosely which extends the width of sandal beyond the warp edge.
Finish: Warp ends tied in one knot at heel
Other: Structural padding on sole

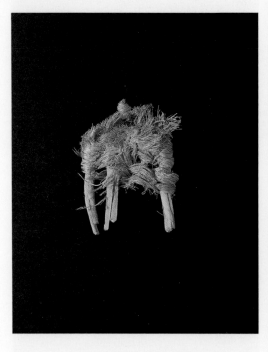

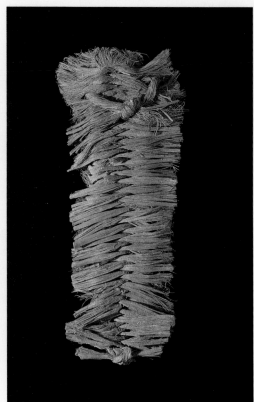

76 *Catalog no.:* 42KA235 (FS13) 23879
Site: Davis Pool Site, Utah
Collector and date: UCRBASP, 1957
Cultural period: Pueblo II-Pueblo III
Construction technique: Plain weave
Dimensions: Length 10.0 cm, width 8.0 cm, depth 1.10 cm
Active elements: Leaf element unspun, cortex intact
Average width: 0.73 cm
Passive elements: Leaf element unspun, cortex intact
Number of passive units: 4
Number in unit: 2
Average width: 0.83 cm
Ties, loops, attachments: Toe: Leaf element looped around middle two warps tied on surface
Shape: Rounded toe, heel missing
Start: Four warps are tied together in one knot.
Body: Over-under plain weave with ends left frayed on sole for padding
Finish: Missing
Other: Structural padding on sole

Catalog no.: 42KA235 AR4008 94.1
Site: Davis Pool Site, Utah
Collector and date: UCRBASP, 1957
Cultural period: Pueblo II-Pueblo III
Construction technique: Plain weave
Dimensions: Length 25.2 cm, width 10.2 cm, depth 1.50 cm
Active elements: Leaf element unspun, cortex intact
Average width: 0.65 cm
Passive elements: Leaf element unspun, cortex intact
Number of passive units: 2
Number in unit: 2(?)
Average width: 0.68 cm
Ties, loops, attachments: Toe: Leaf element looped around warps at toe area and tied in a knot on surface
Shape: Right(?) foot shaping, rounded toe and squared heel
Start: Warps are tied together in one knot at toe. Stitching around knot
Body: Over-under plain weave, beginning with narrow ends of leaf element on top and ending with shredded wide ends on sole for padding. Ends extend beyond body of sandal, increasing width.
Finish: At heel warps are tied in one knot.
Other: Structural padding on sole

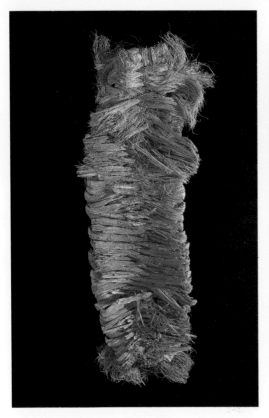

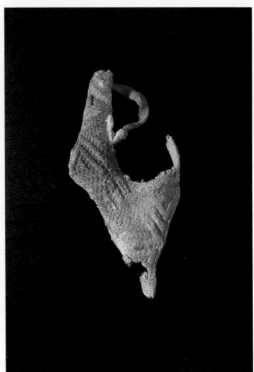

Catalog no.: 42SA598 (89.1) 23985
Site: Defiance House, Utah
Collector and date: UCRBASP, 1959
Cultural period: Pueblo III
Construction technique: Plain weave
Dimensions: Length 25.5 cm, width 9.5 cm, depth
   2.5 cm
Active elements: Leaf element unspun, cortex intact
Average width: 0.61 cm
Passive elements: Leaf element unspun, cortex intact
Number of passive units: 2
Number in unit: 3
Average width: 0.92 cm
Ties, loops, attachments: None apparent
Shape: Left foot shaping, squared toe and rounded
   heel
Start: Warp ends knotted at toe and wrapped with
   five Z twisted shredded leaf elements
Body: Over-under plain weave beginning with
   narrow ends of leaf element on top, ending with
   shredded wide ends on sole for padding. Weft
   elements encircle warps tightly.
Finish: At heel warps are tied in three knots.
Other: Charring on heel warp ends. Structural
   padding on sole.

Catalog no.: 42SA598 (FS47.111) 23985
Site: Defiance House, Utah
Collector and date: UCRBASP, 1959
Cultural period: Pueblo III
Construction technique: Composite
Dimensions: Length 17.0 cm, width 9.4 cm, depth
   0.40 cm
Active elements: Cordage, 2 ply, z-S twist
Average width: 0.10 cm
Passive elements: Cordage, 2 ply, z-S twist
Number of passive units: 31
Number in unit: 1
Average width: 0.12 cm
Ties, loops, attachments: Hide tie wrapped with
   cordage and attached to sandal with knot
Shape: Unknown, fragmentary
Start and Finish: Missing
Body: Raised geometric pattern woven for length of
   fragment

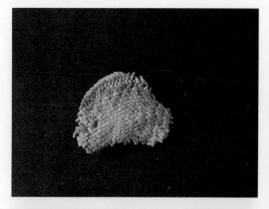

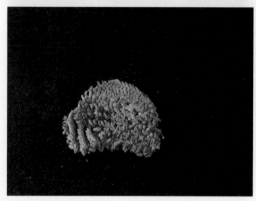

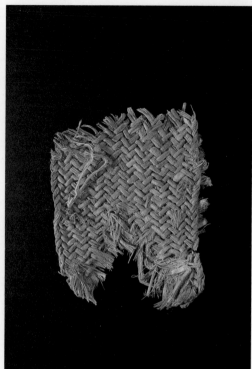

78 *Catalog no.:* 42SA598 (FS69.153) 23985
Site: Defiance House, Utah
Collector and date: UCRBASP, 1959
Cultural period: Pueblo III
Construction technique: Plaited and twined
Dimensions: Length 5.5 cm, width 8.0 cm, depth 8.0 cm
Active elements: Leaf element unspun, cortex intact on surface. Separated leaf elements twisted S and Z on reverse side for raised pattern
Average width: Leaf: 0.34 cm. Twisted: 0.20 cm
Passive elements: N/A
Ties, loops, attachments: None apparent
Shape: Rounded end, fragmentary
Start and Finish: Not determinable
Body: 2/2 twill plaiting with shifts of 1/2. Raised lug pattern on sole appears to be twining with elements twisted S coming from left side and twisted Z when coming from the right side.
Other: Charred

Catalog no.: 42SA598 (FS182.1) 23985
Site: Defiance House, Utah
Collector and date: UCRBASP, 1959
Cultural period: Pueblo III
Construction technique: Plaited
Dimensions: Length 15.0 cm, width 12.0 cm, depth 0.6 cm
Active elements: Leaf element unspun, cortex intact
Average width: 0.49 cm
Passive elements: N/A
Ties, loops, attachments: Edge: Remnant of leaf element loops on both edges. Two possible awl holes.
Shape: Left(?) foot shaping, toe and heel missing, fragmentary
Start and Finish: Missing
Body: 2/2 twill plaiting for length of fragment. Exhausted ends left frayed on sole. No visible shifts
Other: Structural padding on sole

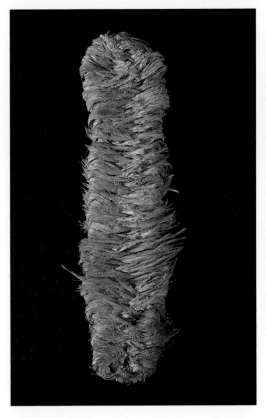

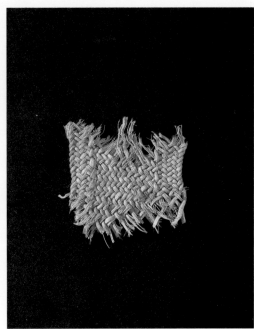

Catalog no.: 936
Site: Double Cave Ruin, Arizona
Collector and date: Byron Cummings, University of
    Utah Expedition, 1909
Cultural period: Unknown
Construction technique: Plain weave
Dimensions: Length 28.0 cm, width 7.0 cm, depth
    1.7 cm
Active elements: Leaf element unspun, cortex intact
Average width: 0.61 cm
Passive elements: Leaf element unspun, cortex intact
Number of passive units: 2
Number in unit: 2
Average width: 0.70 cm
Ties, loops, attachments: Heel: Remnant of cordage 2
    ply, s-Z twist. Edge: Near narrow end appears to
    be an awl(?) hole.
Shape: Rounded toe and heel
Start: Warps tied together at toe in two knots
Body: Over-under plain weave with narrow ends of
    leaf element on top and ending with shredded
    wide ends on sole for padding
Finish: Warps are tied together at heel with two
    knots.
Other: Structural padding on sole

Catalog no.: 937
Site: Double Cave Ruin, Arizona
Collector and date: Byron Cummings, University of
    Utah Expedition, 1909
Cultural period: Unknown
Construction technique: Plaited
Dimensions: Length 5.33 cm, width 8.61 cm, depth
    0.37 cm
Active elements: Leaf element unspun, cortex intact
Average width: 0.30 cm
Passive elements: N/A
Ties, loops, attachments: None apparent
Shape: Unknown, fragmentary
Start and Finish: Missing
Body: 2/2 twill plaiting with shift on both edges
    where every other element crosses parallel
    element and then continues in 2/2 plaiting

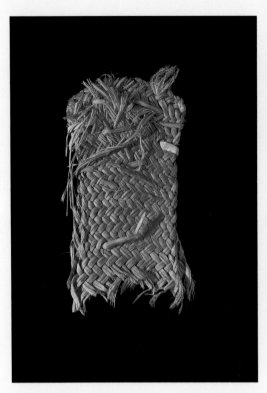
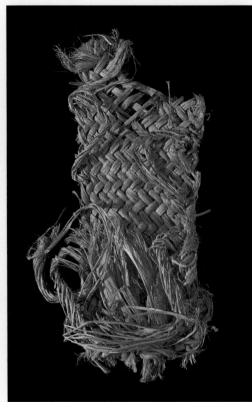

80   *Catalog no.:* 938
Site: Double Cave Ruin, Arizona
Collector and date: Byron Cummings, University of
    Utah Expedition, 1909
Cultural period: Unknown
Construction technique: Plaited
Dimensions: Length 17.0 cm, width 9.2 cm, depth
    0.90 cm
Active elements: Leaf element unspun, cortex intact
Average width: 0.51 cm
Passive elements: N/A
Ties, loops, attachments: Toe: Two long leaf elements
    extend from both sides at toe.
Shape: Squared toe, heel missing
Start: Approximately 20-24 single elements are
    doubled at toe with short ends overlapping in
    pairs.
Body: 2/2 twill plaiting using doubled elements until
    short ends are exhausted. 2/2 plaiting continues
    using single elements. Sandal draws in for
    shaping.
Finish: Missing
Other: Two sandals which appear identical are sewn
    together.

Catalog no.: 939
Site: Double Cave Ruin, Arizona
Collector and date: Byron Cummings, University of
    Utah Expedition, 1909
Cultural period: Unknown
Construction technique: Plaited
Dimensions: Length 26.0 cm, width 9.6 cm, depth
    0.87 cm
Active elements: Leaf element unspun, cortex intact
Average width: 0.59 cm
Passive elements: N/A
Ties, loops, attachments: Toe: Leaf element loops
    from left toe area stitching into body of sandal at
    edge. Heel: Leaf elements tie across heel. Edge:
    Leaf elements on both edges loop and stitch into
    sandal. Knot at each edge
Shape: Squared heel, toe area missing on right side
Start: Approximately 20-22 elements are doubled at
    toe with short ends overlapping in pairs.
Body: 2/2 twill plaiting using doubled elements until
    short ends are exhausted. 2/2 plaiting continues
    using single elements for length of sandal. One
    element dropped near heel for shaping
Finish: At heel edge element forms a transverse bar
    over which one half the elements are folded
    with ends protruding on upper surface. The
    other half of the elements are cut short at heel
    edge. Stitching at heel edge after completion of
    sandal

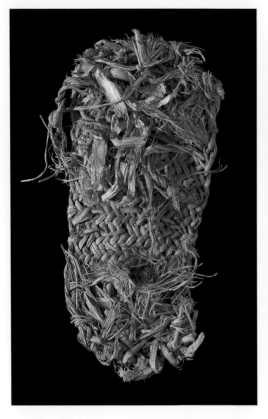
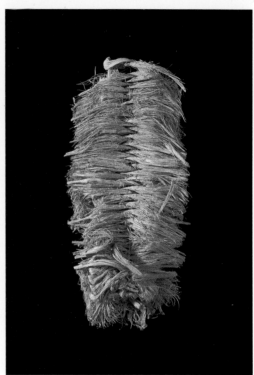

Catalog no.: 940
Site: Double Cave Ruin, Arizona
Collector and date: Byron Cummings, University of
  Utah Expedition, 1909
Cultural period: Unknown
Construction technique: Plaited
Dimensions: Length 25.42 cm, width 12.13 cm,
  depth 0.95 cm
Active elements: Leaf element unspun, cortex intact
Average width: 0.54 cm
Passive elements: N/A
Ties, loops, attachments: Toe: Leaf element ties and
  loop twisted S. Heel: Remnants of ties, one knot,
  leaf element twisted S. Edge: Cordage loop 2 ply,
  s-Z twist
Shape: Rounded toe and squared heel
Start: Active elements folded at toe
Body: 2/2 twill plaiting for length of sandal. Two
  horizontal rows of stitching appear at
  midsection. Exhausted ends frayed on sole
Finish: At heel a horizontal transverse element is
  knotted in a loop. Terminal elements are
  wrapped around the top transverse bar to the
  upper surface and bottom bar to the sole.
Other: Structural padding on sole

Catalog no.: 42SA377 (FS50.1) 23988
Site: Fence Ruin, Utah
Collector and date: UCRBSP, 1959
Cultural period: Pueblo II-Pueblo III
Construction technique: Plain weave
Dimensions: Length 20.0 cm, width 9.47 cm, depth
  1.51 cm
Active elements: Leaf element unspun, cortex intact
Average width: 5.7 cm
Passive elements: Leaf element unspun, cortex intact
Number of passive units: 2
Number in unit: 1
Average width: 0.87 cm
Ties, loops, attachments: None apparent
Shape: Rounded toe and heel, toe end fragmentary
Start: Toe end incomplete
Body: Over-under plain weave beginning with
  narrow ends of leaf element on top and ending
  with shredded wide ends on sole for padding.
  Ends extend beyond body of sandal.
Finish: At heel, warps ended with three knots
Other: Structural padding on sole

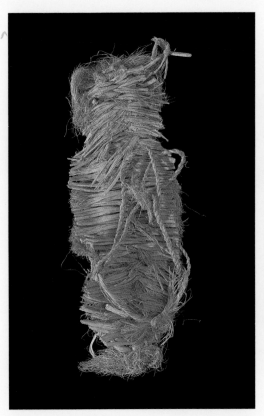

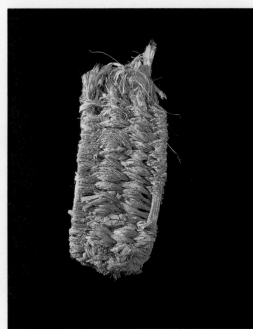

Catalog no.: 42SA619 (FS26.246) 24046
Site: Gourd House, Utah
Collector and date: UCRBASP 1960
Cultural period: Pueblo I-Pueblo III
Construction technique: Plain weave
Dimensions: Length 27.0 cm, width 10.00 cm, depth
1.34 cm
Active elements: Leaf element unspun, cortex intact
Average width: 0.60 cm
Passive elements: Leaf elements unspun, cortex
intact
Number of passive units: 2
Number in unit: 2
Average width: 0.70 cm
Ties, loops, attachments: Toe: Remnant of toe loop,
passed under sole and knotted on top. Heel:
Loop passed under sole and knotted on top: tie
has S twist. A length of cordage, 2 ply s-Z, is
looped around both sides of heel loop, laced
down toward end. Ends are knotted together.
Shape: Rounded toe and heel
Start: Warps are tied together at toe in two knots.
Body: Over-under plain weave beginning with
narrow ends of leaf element on top and ending
with shredded wide ends on sole for padding.
Ends extend beyond body of sandal.
Finish: At heel warps are tied into 2 knots, one in
front of the other.
Other: Structural padding on sole

Catalog no.: 42KA443 (FS12.6) 23906
Site: Hermitage Site, Utah
Collector and date: UCRBASP 1958
Cultural period: Pueblo II-Pueblo III
Construction technique: Plain weave
Dimensions: Length 16 cm, width 7.0 cm, depth 1.0
cm
Active elements: Leaf element, unspun, cortex intact
Average width: 0.55 cm
Passive elements: Leaf element unspun, cortex intact
Number of passive units: 4
Number in unit: 1
Average width: 0.6 cm
Ties, loops, attachments: Remnant of heel tie(?)
Shape: Unknown, fragmentary
Start: Missing
Body: Tightly packed plain weave continues to heel
with wefts slightly twisted S.
Finish: At the heel warp ends appear split and
wrapped around an adjacent warp split end with
ends tucked into the sandal, creating a braided-
like effect across the heel.
Other: Some structural padding on sole

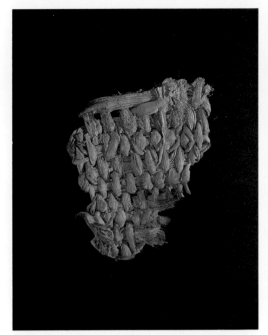
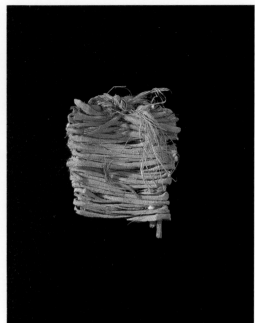

Catalog no.: 42KA443 (FS13.13) 23906
Site: Hermitage Site, Utah
Collector and date: UCRBASP, 1958
Cultural period: Pueblo II-Pueblo III
Construction technique: Plain weave
Dimensions: Length 12.7 cm, width 11.4 cm, depth 0.90 cm
Active elements: Leaf element, unspun, cortex intact
Average width: 1.04 cm
Passive elements: Leaf element unspun, cortex intact
Number of passive units: 18
Number in unit: 1
Average width: 0.70 cm
Ties, loops, attachments: None apparent
Shape: Unknown, fragmentary
Start: Missing
Body: Over-under plain weave with warps set close together and weft pulled tightly each row to form a warp-faced weave with warps predominating
Finish: Missing

Catalog no.: 42KA443 (FS18.17) 23906
Site: Hermitage Site, Utah
Collector and date: UCRBASP 1958
Cultural period: Pueblo II-Pueblo III
Construction technique: Plain weave
Dimensions: Length 9.50 cm, width 9.00 cm, depth 1.50 cm
Active elements: Leaf element unspun, cortex intact
Average width: 0.42 cm
Passive elements: Leaf elements unspun, cortex intact
Number of passive units: 2
Number in unit: 2
Average width: 0.75 cm
Ties, loops, attachments: None apparent
Shape: Fragmentary; one end of sandal is missing.
Start or Finish: Four warps are tied together in one knot at toe which is broken on one side.
Body: Over-under plain weave beginning with narrow ends of leaf element on top and ending with shredded wide ends on sole for padding
Other: Numerous cotton-like balls cling to upper and lower sides of sandal. Structural padding on sole

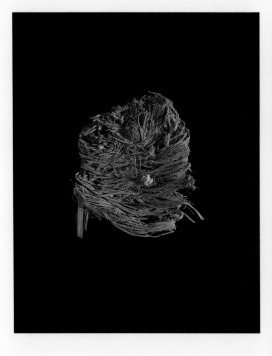
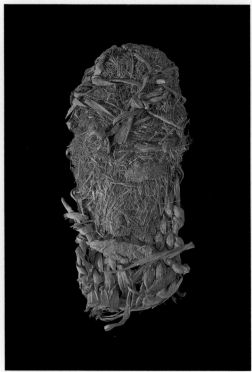

Catalog no.: 42KA443 (FS19.1) 23906
Site: Hermitage Site, Utah
Collector and date: UCRBASP, 1958
Cultural period: Pueblo II-Pueblo III
Construction technique: Plain weave
Dimensions: Length 22.2 cm, width 11.2 cm, depth 2.7 cm
Active elements: Leaf element unspun, cortex intact
Average width: 0.71 cm
Passive elements: Leaf element unspun, cortex intact
Number of passive units: 15
Number in unit: 2
Average width: 0.64 cm
Ties, loops, attachments: Toe and edge have 6-7 areas where wefts loop and knot around warp elements and then are laced together on top of padded toe area in three separate square knots.
Shape: Left(?) foot shaping, rounded toe and heel
Start: Warps are folded over first weft element.
Body: 1/1 plain weave for length of sandal, with warps set close together and weft pulled tightly each row to form warp faced weave with warps predominating
Finish: Terminating weft element drawn across heel, not engaging warps then knotted and tucked back into warp/weft crossing. Warps are cut.
Other: Heavy padding of Poaceae leaf on upper 2/3 of sandal

84 Catalog no.: 42KA443 (FS18.19) 23906
Site: Hermitage Site, Utah
Collector and date: UCRBASP, 1958
Cultural period: Pueblo II-Pueblo III
Construction technique: Plain weave
Dimensions: Length 11.00 cm, width 9.00 cm, depth 2.00 cm
Active elements: Shredded leaf elements, unspun, cortex intact
Average width: 0.76 cm
Passive elements: Leaf element, unspun, cortex intact
Number of passive units: 2
Number in unit: ?
Average width: 0.65 cm
Ties, loops, attachments: Remnants of a knot or loop near toe(?) end of sandal
Shape: Fragmentary
Start: Unable to determine
Body: Over-under plain weave ending with leaf elements shredded on sole for padding
Finish: Unable to determine
Other: Structural padding on sole

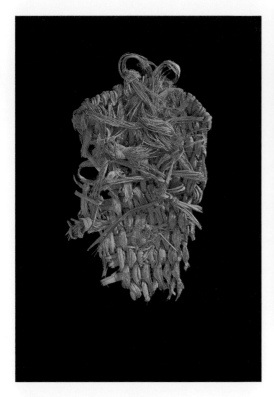

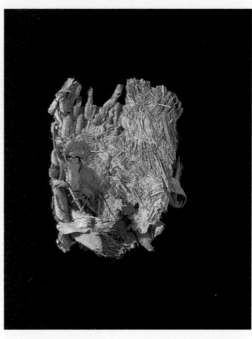

Catalog no.: 42KA443 (FS19.2) 23906
Site: Hermitage Site, Utah
Collector and date: UCRBASP 1958
Cultural period: Pueblo II-Pueblo III
Construction technique: Plain weave
Dimensions: Length 19.9 cm, width 11.6 cm, depth 1.0 cm
Active elements: Leaf element unspun, cortex intact
Average width: 0.80 cm
Passive elements: Leaf element unspun, cortex intact
Number of passive units: 16
Number in unit: 1
Average width: 0.42 cm
Ties, loops, attachments: Toe and Edge: Loops are attached to warp and weft then tied across upper surface of sandal in square knots.
Shape: Rounded toe, missing heel
Start: Eight warps are folded at toe over first weft to form 16 warps.
Body: Over-under plain weave for body of sandal with warps set close together and wefts pulled tightly each row creating a warp faced weave structure
Finish: Missing

Catalog no.: 42KA443 (FS19.3) 23906
Site: Hermitage Site, Utah
Collector and date: UCRBASP, 1958
Cultural period: Pueblo II-Pueblo III
Construction technique: Plain weave
Dimensions: Length 15.5 cm, width 13.1 cm, depth 1.84 cm
Active elements: Leaf element unspun, cortex intact
Average width: 0.60 cm
Passive elements: Leaf elements unspun, cortex intact
Number of passive units: ?
Number in unit: ?
Average width: 0.62 cm
Ties, loops, attachments: None apparent
Shape: Toe missing, heel area rounded
Start: Missing
Body: Over-under plain weave with warps set close together and weft pulled tightly each row to form a warp faced weave structure
Finish: Missing
Other: Both surfaces caked with mud but upper surface has grass(?) mixed in which might have been padding.

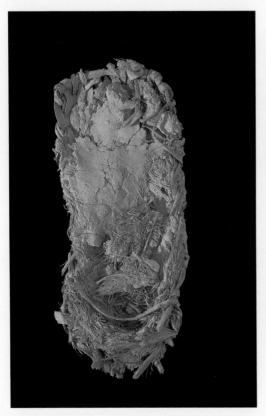

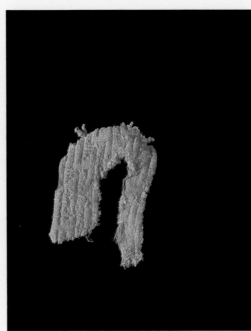

86　*Catalog no.:* 42KA443 (FS24) 23906
Site: Hermitage Site, Utah
Collector and date: UCRBASP, 1958
Cultural period: Pueblo II-Pueblo III
Construction technique: Plain weave
Dimensions: Length 25.5 cm, width 11.5 cm, depth 2.1 cm
Active elements: Leaf element unspun, cortex intact
Average width: 0.62 cm
Passive elements: Leaf element unspun, cortex intact
Number of passive units: 20
Number in unit: ?
Average width: 0.61 cm
Ties, loops, attachments: Toe: Leaf element knotted to warp at toe and looped around warp at edge. Heel: Long loop fragment
Shape: Right(?) foot shaping, slightly rounded toe and round cupped heel
Start: Warps folded over first weft element
Body: 1/1 plain weave for length of sandal with warps set close together and weft pulled tightly each row to form a warp faced weave with warps predominating
Finish: At heel it appears warp ends are left protruding with wefts pulled tight to produce cupped heel.
Other: Caking with mud and grass(?) on inside of sandal

Catalog no.: 623
Site: Hostien Canyon, Arizona
Collector and date: Byron Cummings, University of Utah Expedition, 1909
Cultural period: Basketmaker III
Construction technique: Composite
Dimensions: Length 10.8 cm, width 7.5 cm, depth 0.47 cm
Active elements: Cordage, 2 ply, z-S twist
Average width: 0.14 cm
Passive elements: Cordage, 2 ply, z-S twist
Number of passive units: 28
Number in unit: 1
Average width: 0.15 cm
Ties, loops, attachments: None apparent
Shape: Unknown, fragmentary
Start and Finish: Missing
Body: Fragment section woven in raised geometric pattern

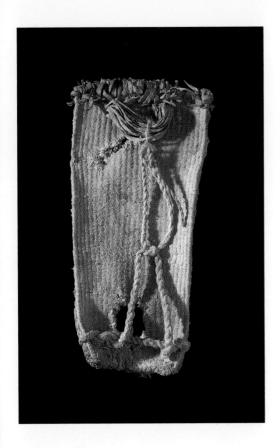

Catalog no.: 624
Site: Hostien Canyon, Arizona
Collector and date: Byron Cummings, University of
    Utah Expedition, 1909
Cultural period: Basketmaker II
Construction technique: Composite
Dimensions: Length 23.2 cm, width 11.0 cm, depth
    0.70 cm
Active elements: Cordage, 2 ply, z-S twist
Average width: 0.15 cm
Passive elements: Cordage, 3 ply, s-Z twist
Number of passive units: 28
Number in unit: 1
Average width: 0.22 cm
Ties, loops, attachments: Toe: Nine strips of hide are
    sewn across middle toe area as loops. Cordage,
    2 ply s-Z twist, loops around toe strips and is
    knotted at instep to heel loop. Heel: Cord, 2 ply
    s-Z twist, loops and stitches into sandal at both
    edges and is knotted to instep loop.
Shape: Squared toe and heel

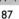

Start: At toe it appears 14 elements were folded
    over a rigid element secured from two points.
    Fiber is added to toe for bulk then wrapped
    with hide across entire toe area.
Body: The sole has the appearance of two layers
    and only one where raised pattern has worn. It
    appears there were 3-4 rows of plain weave
    selvage to selvage, followed by a row of two
    element weft wrapping which went back and
    forth across the sole but did not connect to side
    selvages.
Finish: Warp ends stitched alternately to surface
    and to sole, where they are clipped short
Other: Red ocher(?) stain on sole of heel. Fringing
    at toe may have been structural or due to wear.

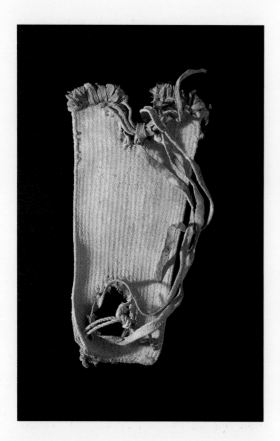

2 ply z twist (each ply 2 ply, z-S twist) with a
square knot.

88   *Catalog no.:* 625

Site: Hostien Canyon, Arizona

Collector and date: Byron Cummings, University of
    Utah Expedition, 1909

Cultural period: Basketmaker II

Construction technique: Composite

Dimensions: Length 22.0 cm, width 10.0 cm, depth
    0.56 cm

Active elements: Cordage, 2 ply, z-S twist

Average width: 0.13 cm

Passive elements: Cordage, 3 ply, s-Z twist

Number of passive units: 28

Number in unit: 1

Average width: 0.27 cm

Ties, loops, attachments: Toe: Five(?) hide strips are
    sewn across middle of toe area. Hide tie is
    knotted to middle of strips and extends to heel
    loop, where it is sewn with a piece of cord (2
    ply, s-Z twist) to another piece of hide that
    extends back to toe, loops around toe loop and
    is sewn to another piece of hide. Heel: Two hide
    ties from right side are connected to 2 cord ties,

Shape: Squared toe and heel

Start: At toe it appears 14 elements were folded
    over a rigid element secured from two points.
    There is one row of twining using hair on
    surface only. Fiber is added to toe and then
    wrapped with hide across entire toe area.

Body: The sole has the appearance of two layers
    and only one where raised pattern has worn. It
    appears there were 3-4 rows of plain weave
    selvage to selvage, followed by a row of two-
    element weft wrapping which went back and
    forth across the sole but did not connect to side
    selvages.

Finish: Warp ends stitched alternately to surface
    and to sole, where they are clipped short

Other: Fringing at toe may have been structural or
    due to wear.

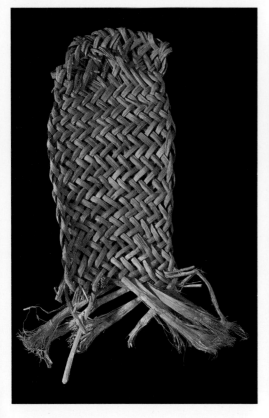
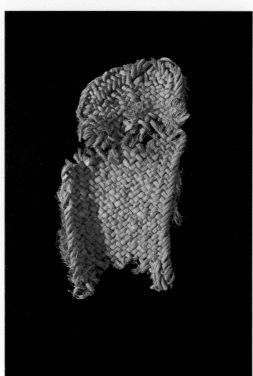

Catalog no.: 2562
Site: Inscription House, Arizona
Collector and date: Byron Cummings, University of Utah Expedition, 1914
Cultural period: Basketmaker III-Pueblo III
Construction technique: Plaited
Dimensions: Length 27.0 cm, width 10.0 cm, depth 0.45 cm
Active elements: Leaf element unspun, cortex intact
Average width: 0.47 cm
Passive elements: N/A
Ties, loops, attachments: None apparent
Shape: Left foot shaping, rounded toe with jog, heel incomplete
Start: Twenty-one elements fold at toe with narrow ends overlapping for a short distance. Five additional elements are folded for toe jog.
Body: 2/2 twill plaiting with shift of 2/3/2 near heel where two elements are dropped with ends left protruding on sole
Finish: Incomplete

Catalog no.: 42SA738 (FS10.1) 24072
Site: Ivy Shelter, Utah
Collector and date: UCRBASP, 1962
Cultural period: Pueblo III
Construction technique: Plaited
Dimensions: Length 18.0 cm, width 8.70 cm, depth 0.90 cm
Active elements: Leaf element unspun, cortex intact
Average width: 0.36 cm
Passive elements: N/A
Ties, loops, attachments: Toe: One possible remnant at middle of toe
Shape: Left foot shaping, tapered toe, heel missing
Start: Active elements folded at toe
Body: 2/2 twill plaiting with edges pulled in tightly. Ends left frayed on sole
Finish: Missing
Other: Structural padding on sole

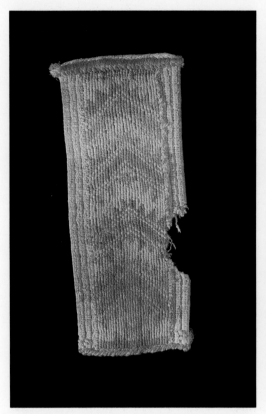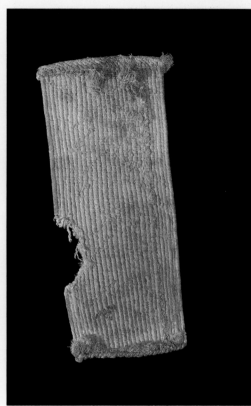

90   *Catalog no.:* 8093
Site: Kanab Canyon, Utah
Collector and date: James Little, Kanab, Utah, 1923
Cultural period: Basketmaker II(?)
Construction technique: Composite
Dimensions: Length 25.25 cm, width 10.75 cm, depth 0.30 cm
Active elements: Cordage, 2 ply, z-S twist
Average width: 0.13 cm
Passive elements: Cordage, 3 ply, z-S twist
Number of passive units: 28 .
Number in unit: 1
Average width: 0.30 cm
Ties, loops, attachments: Toe: Four remnant stitches, 2 ply, s-Z twist. Heel: Four remnant stitches 2 ply, s-Z twist
Shape: Squared toe and heel
Start: At toe it appears 14 elements were folded over a rigid element secured from two points. Braided selvages on both edges of toe. One row of twining on sole at toe between 2 rows of darker twined stitches. Dark yucca braid on surface only
Body: 1/1 plain weave with warp wrapping every other row. Six warps on both sides carry only natural color wefts and wrap around warp, making an extra twist between warps to create a knot appearance. Center panel with red and blue dyed wefts appears to be added weft elements that begin and end on surface where ends are evident. Because the number of vertical ridges in central panel is doubled, there is a second layer of warps which are a fine 2 ply cordage. Dyed wefts wrap around these warps twice before progressing to the next fine warp. Rows of natural color plain weave continue and probably lock added warps in place.
Finish: At heel there is one row of twining for center panel. Warp ends are folded over adjacent warps, alternating with surface and sole, and clipped.
Other: Reverse side has a faded diagonal design painted in red.

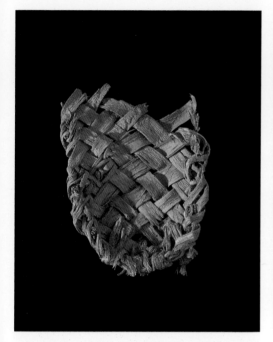
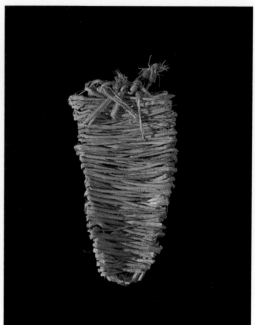

Catalog no.: 23967
Site: Lavender Canyon, San Juan County, Utah
Collector and date: Bates Wilson, 1956
Cultural period: Unknown
Construction technique: Plaited
Dimensions: Length 15.5 cm, width 11.0 cm, depth 0.54 cm
Active elements: Leaf element unspun, cortex intact
Average width: 1.32 cm
Passive elements: N/A
Ties, loops, attachments: Stitching on both sides for possible attachments
Shape: Round cupped heel, toe missing
Start: Missing
Body: 1/1 plaiting for length of fragment
Finish: Ends wrapped over a transverse element with ends protruding
Other: Stitching on both sides toward heel

Catalog no.: 42KA276 (FS12.1) 23905
Site: Lizard Alcove, Utah
Collector and date: UCRBASP, 1958
Cultural period: Pueblo II-Pueblo III
Construction technique: Plain weave
Dimensions: Length 15.5 cm, width 7.5 cm, depth 0.9 cm
Active elements: Leaf element unspun, cortex intact
Average width: 0.41 cm
Passive elements: Leaf element unspun, cortex intact
Number of passive units: 2
Number in unit: 3(?)
Average width: 0.72 cm
Ties, loops, attachments: One knot near heel
Shape: Squared toe and rounded heel
Start: Two warp units of three(?) warps each are divided and tied together at toe in approximately four knots.
Body: Over-under plain weave with shredded ends on sole for padding
Finish: At heel remains of one knot visible
Other: Structural padding on sole

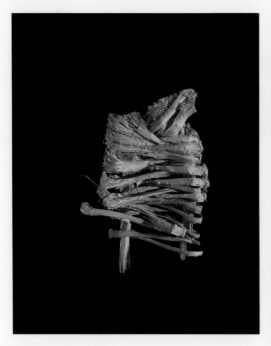
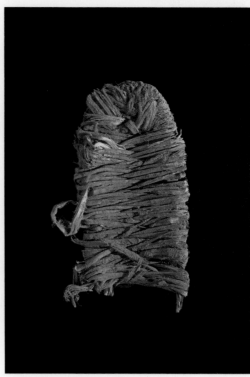

92   *Catalog no.:* 42KA276 (FS41.1) 23905
Site: Lizard Alcove, Utah
Collector and date: UCRBASP, 1958
Cultural period: Pueblo II-Pueblo III
Construction technique: Plain weave
Dimensions: Length 13.5 cm, width 8.0 cm, depth
  1.4 cm
Active elements: Leaf element unspun, cortex intact
Average width: 0.60 cm
Passive elements: Leaf element unspun, cortex intact
Number of passive units: 2
Number in unit: 1
Average width: 0.80 cm
Ties, loops, attachments: None apparent
Shape: Toe and heel missing
Start: Missing
Body: Over-under plain weave with ends shredded
  on sole for padding
Finish: Possible remains of one knot at heel or toe
Other: Structural padding on sole

Catalog no.: 42KA276 (FS41.2) 23905
Site: Lizard Alcove, Utah
Collector and date: UCRBASP, 1958
Cultural period: Pueblo II-Pueblo III
Construction technique: Plain weave
Dimensions: Length 15.8 cm, width 8.5 cm, depth
  1.4 cm
Active elements: Leaf element unspun, cortex intact
Average width: 0.34 cm
Passive elements: Leaf element unspun, cortex intact
Number of passive units: 2
Number in unit: 1
Average width: 0.82 cm
Ties, loops, attachments: Edge: Remnants of 2 loops
  for lacing along one edge
Shape: Rounded toe, heel missing
Start: Warps are tied in one knot with weft
  wrapping over knot.
Body: Over-under plain weave with shredded ends
  on sole for padding
Finish: Missing
Other: Structural padding on sole

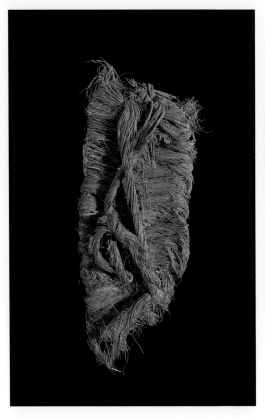

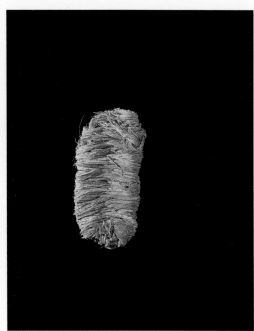

Catalog no.: 42KA276 (FS63.2) 23905
Site: Lizard Alcove, Utah
Collector and date: UCRBASP, 1958
Cultural period: Pueblo II-Pueblo III
Construction technique: Plain weave
Dimensions: Length 20 cm, width 8.5 cm, depth 1.4 cm
Active elements: Leaf element unspun, cortex intact
Average width: 0.72 cm
Passive elements: Leaf element unspun, cortex intact
Number of passive units: 2
Number in unit: 1
Average width: 0.92 cm
Ties, loops, attachments: Toe: Leaf element loop, S twist. Heel: Two ties Z twisted extend from heel to toe loop where they are knotted together.
Shape: Rounded toe and squared heel
Start: Knotted start with two warps tied together at toe in one knot
Body: Over-under plain weave with shredded ends on sole for padding
Finish: At heel are two warp knots.
Other: Structural padding on sole

Catalog no.: 42KA276 (FS66.15) 23905
Site: Lizard Alcove, Utah
Collector and date: UCRBASP, 1958
Cultural period: Pueblo II-Pueblo III
Construction technique: Plain weave
Dimensions: Length 10.5 cm, width 5.2 cm, depth 0.85 cm
Active elements: Leaf element unspun, cortex intact
Average width: 0.36 cm
Passive elements: Leaf element unspun, cortex intact
Number of passive units: 2
Number in unit: 1
Average width: 0.68 cm
Ties, loops, attachments: Edge: Remnants of tie on one edge near one end, knotted into sole
Shape: A small child(?) size sandal, rounded at finished end
Start or Finish: Warp elements knotted together
Body: Over-under plain weave with shredded ends on sole for padding
Other: Structural padding on sole

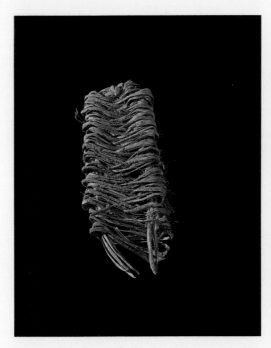 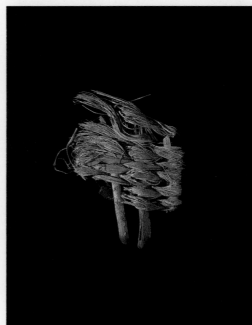

94　*Catalog no.:* 42KA276 (FS66.2) 23905
Site: Lizard Alcove, Utah
Collector and date: UCRBASP, 1958
Cultural period: Pueblo II-Pueblo III
Construction technique: Plain weave
Dimensions: Length 15.2 cm, width 7.0 cm, depth
　1.5 cm
Active elements: Leaf element unspun, cortex intact
Average width: 0.39 cm
Passive elements: Leaf element unspun, cortex intact
Number of passive units: 2
Number in unit: 1
Average width: 0.71 cm
Ties, loops, attachments: None
Shape: Rounded finished end
Start or Finish: Warps are knotted together.
Body: Over-under plain weave with shredded ends
　on sole for padding
Other: Structural padding on sole

Catalog no.: 42KA276 (FS66.53) 23905
Site: Lizard Alcove, Utah
Collector and date: UCRBASP, 1958
Cultural period: Pueblo II-Pueblo III
Construction technique: Plain weave
Dimensions: Length 10.0 cm, width 9.0 cm, depth
　0.90 cm
Active elements: Leaf element unspun, cortex intact
Average width: 0.86 cm
Passive elements: Leaf element unspun, cortex intact
Number of passive units: 4
Number in unit: 1
Average width: 0.94 cm
Ties, loops, attachments: None apparent
Shape: Fragmentary
Start or Finish: Missing
Body: Over-under plain weave for length of
　fragment

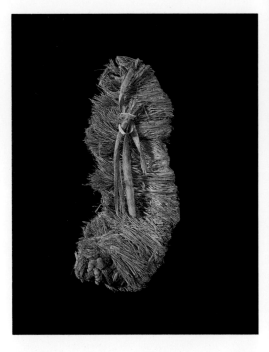

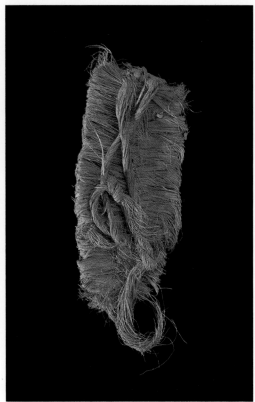

Catalog no.: 42KA276 (FS69.2) 23905
Site: Lizard Alcove, Utah
Collector and date: UCRBASP, 1958
Cultural period: Pueblo II-Pueblo III
Construction technique: Plain weave
Dimensions: Length 18 cm, width 6.5 cm, depth 1.3 cm
Active elements: Leaf element unspun, cortex intact
Average width: Unable to determine; too shredded
Passive elements: Leaf element unspun, cortex intact
Number of passive units: 2
Number in unit: 2(?)
Average width: 0.96 cm
Ties, loops, attachments: Remnants of an attachment on top of sandal
Shape: Rounded toe and heel
Start: Warps are tied together in one knot at toe.
Body: Over-under plain weave with shredded ends left on sole for padding
Finish: Four warp knots at heel
Other: Structural padding on sole

Catalog no.: 42KA276 (FS69.3) 23905
Site: Lizard Alcove, Utah
Collector and date: UCRBSP, 1958
Cultural period: Pueblo II-Pueblo III
Construction technique: Plain weave
Dimensions: Length 20.00 cm, width 9.20 cm, depth 1.40 cm
Active elements: Leaf elements unspun, cortex intact
Average width: 0.55 cm
Passive elements: Leaf elements unspun, cortex intact
Number of passive units: 4
Number in unit: 3 or 4
Average width: 1.00 cm
Ties, loops, attachments: Edge: Shredded leaf element loop (Z twist) remains on one side of sandal unattached but looped around a piece of cordage that extends from the body of the sandal through the middle of the loop and ends in a square knot.
Shape: Fragmentary
Start or Finish: Each warp is wrapped around adjacent warp and frayed to form padding beyond the end of sandal.
Body: Over-under plain weave beginning and ending on sole where ends are shredded for padding
Other: Structural padding on sole

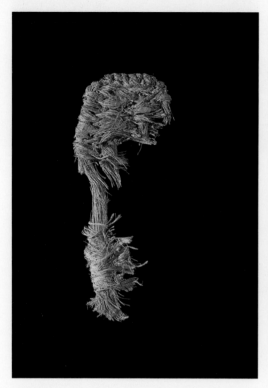 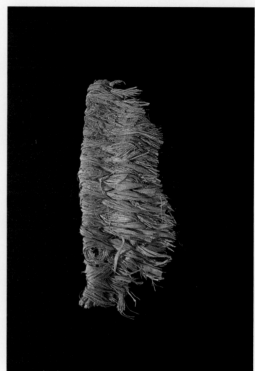

96 *Catalog no.:* 42KA276 (FS69.4) 23905
Site: Lizard Alcove, Utah
Collector and date: UCRBSP, 1958
Cultural period: Pueblo II-Pueblo III
Construction technique: Plain weave
Dimensions: Length 20.5 cm, width 8.0 cm, depth
    1.0 cm
Active elements: Shredded leaf element unspun,
    cortex intact
Average width: 0.5 cm
Passive elements: Shredded leaf element, twisted S
Number of passive units: 4
Number in unit: 1(?)
Average width: 0.73 cm
Ties, loops, attachments: None apparent
Shape: Rounded end, fragmentary
Start or Finish: Ends appear knotted twice and cut
    close. There appears to be one row of twining
    below knots.
Body: Over-under plain weave for length of
    fragment

Catalog no.: 42KA276 (FS69.5) 23905
Site: Lizard Alcove, Utah
Collector and date: UCRBASP, 1958
Cultural period: Pueblo II-Pueblo III
Construction technique: Plain weave
Dimensions: Length 18.5 cm, width 7.5 cm, depth
    0.9 cm
Active elements: Leaf element unspun, cortex intact
Average width: 0.64 cm
Passive elements: Leaf element unspun, cortex intact
Number of passive units: ?
Number in unit: 1
Average width: 0.75 cm
Ties, loops, attachments: None apparent
Shape: Fragmentary
Start: Missing
Body: Over-under plain weave
Finish: One knot visible at heel(?) or toe (?)

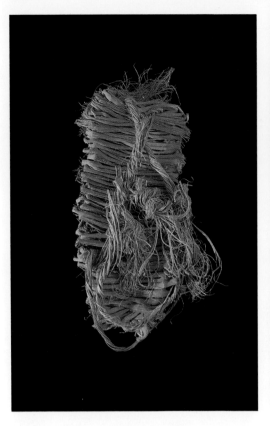
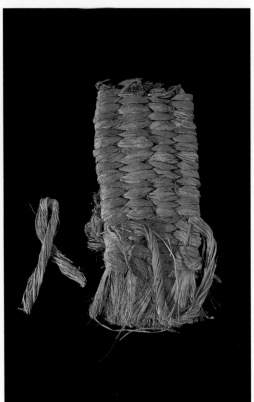

Catalog no.: 42KA276 (FS71.1) 23905
Site: Lizard Alcove, Utah
Collector and date: UCRBASP, 1958
Cultural period: Pueblo II-Pueblo III
Construction technique: Plain weave
Dimensions: Length 19.5 cm, width 9.5 cm, depth 3.5 cm
Active elements: Leaf element unspun, cortex intact
Average width: 0.51 cm
Passive elements: Leaf element unspun, cortex intact
Number of passive units: 2
Number in unit: 2
Average width: 0.50 cm
Ties, loops, attachments: Toe and Edge: Two ties, twisted S, emerge at middle of toe as extensions of warp. They cross at toe and extend to edges near heel where they loop through wefts. Each goes around ankle in opposite directions and is left as a loose tie knotted at end.
Shape: Toe and heel appear rounded.
Start: Two warps are tied at toe with ends extending for ties.
Body: Over-under, plain weave beginning with narrow end of leaf element on top and ending with shredded wide ends on sole for padding
Finish: Warps are knotted at heel.
Other: Structural padding on sole

Catalog no.: 42KA276 (FS72) 23905
Site: Lizard Alcove, Utah
Collector and date: UCRBASP, 1958
Cultural period: Pueblo II-Pueblo III
Construction technique: Plain weave
Dimensions: Length 20.5 cm, width 9.0 cm, depth 1.4 cm
Active elements: Leaf element unspun, cortex intact
Average width: 0.66 cm
Passive elements: Leaf element unspun, cortex intact
Number of passive units: 4
Number in unit: 1
Average width: 0.96 cm
Ties, loops, attachments: Heel: Loop, S twist attached at heel
Shape: Toe missing. Heel squared with splayed warp ends protruding for 4.0 cm
Start: Missing
Body: Over-under plain weave from toe to heel
Finish: At heel splayed warps extend for 4.0 cm.

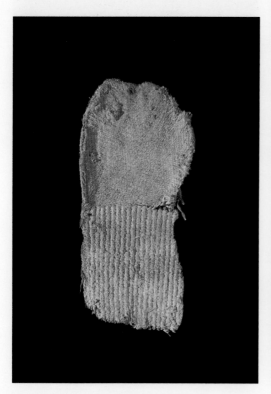

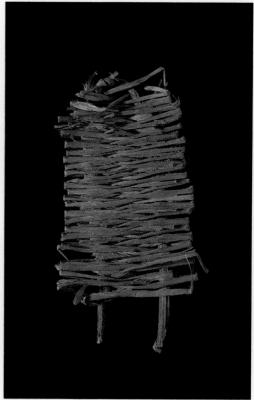

Catalog no.: 7899
Site: Moki Canyon, Utah
Collector and date: University of Utah Expedition, San Juan County, 1926
Cultural period: Basketmaker III(?)
Construction technique: Composite
Dimensions: Length 19.3 cm, width 9.3 cm, depth 0.83 cm
Active elements: Cordage, 2 ply, z-S twist
Average width: 0.10 cm
Passive elements: Cordage, 3 ply, z-S twist
Number of passive units: 20
Number in unit: 1 (except where doubled at toe)
Average width: 0.18 cm
Ties, loops, attachments: Toe: Four remnant plugs visible on left side and two on right side. Edge: Three sets of plugs along left edge. One plug left near heel corner.
Shape: Right foot shaping, scalloped toe, heel missing
Start: Scalloped toe start
Body: 2/2 alternate pair twining over doubled warps for forward one-third section of sandal at which point doubled warps end. Rear section of sandal appears to be twining (possibly 3 element) and wrapping combined with several rows of twining.
Finish: Missing

Catalog no.: 2534
Site: Monument Park, Utah
Collector and date: Byron Cummings, University of Utah Expedition, 1914
Cultural period: Pueblo III
Construction technique: Plain weave
Dimensions: Length 21.0 cm, width 10.0 cm, depth 0.7 cm
Active elements: Leaf element unspun, cortex intact
Average width: 0.49 cm
Passive elements: Leaf element unspun, cortex intact
Number of passive units: 2
Number in unit: 2
Average width: 0.70 cm
Ties, loops, attachments: None apparent
Shape: Unknown
Start or Finish: Warps are tied together at one end in a knot. Opposite end broken
Body: Over-under plain weave beginning with narrow end of leaf element on top near center, and ending with shredded wide ends on sole for padding. Weft elements encircle warps both tightly and loosely which extends the width of sandal beyond the warp edge.
Other: Structural padding on sole

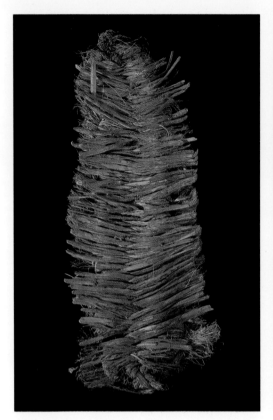

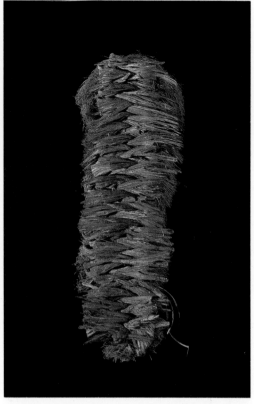

Catalog no.: 2535
Site: Monument Park, Utah
Collector and date: Byron Cummings, University of
Utah Expedition, 1914
Cultural period: Pueblo III
Construction technique: Plain weave
Dimensions: Length 27.5 cm, width 10.2 cm, depth
2.02 cm
Active elements: Leaf element unspun, cortex intact
Average width: 0.53 cm
Passive elements: Leaf element unspun, cortex intact
Number of passive units: 2
Number in unit: 3
Average width: 0.44 cm
Ties, loops, attachments: None apparent
Shape: Rounded toe and heel
Start: Warps are tied together in two knots at toe.
Body: Over-under plain weave beginning with
narrow end of leaf element on top and ending
with shredded wide ends on sole for padding.
Short wefts encircle warps tightly but end on
surface and on sole extend beyond body of
sandal, increasing width.
Other: Structural padding on sole

Catalog no.: 2565
Site: Monument Park, Utah
Collector and date: Byron Cummings, University of
Utah Expedition, 1914
Cultural period: Pueblo III
Construction technique: Plain weave
Dimensions: Length 23.50 cm, width 7.72 cm, depth
0.75 cm
Active elements: Leaf element unspun, cortex intact
Average width: 0.48 cm
Passive elements: Leaf element unspun, cortex intact
Number of passive units: 2
Number in unit: 3
Average width: 1.50 cm
Ties, loops, attachments: Leaf element woven under
warp, over wefts and under opposite warp near
knotted end of sandal
Shape: Rounded end, opposite end broken
Start or Finish: Warps are tied together at one end
in three separate knots.
Body: Over-under plain weave beginning with
narrow ends of leaf element on top and ending
with shredded wide ends on sole for padding.
Ends extend beyond warp edge.
Other: Structural padding on sole

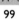

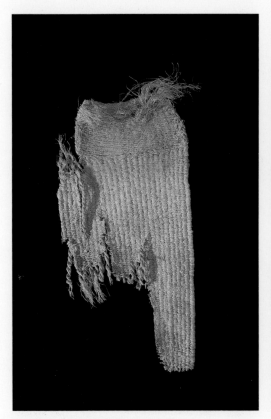
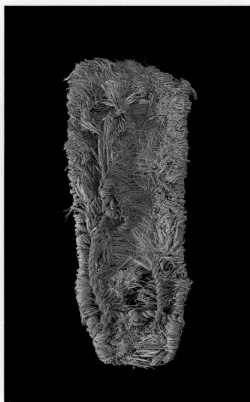

100   *Catalog no.:* 2606
Site: Monument Park, Utah
Collector and date: Byron Cummings, University of
   Utah Expedition, 1914
Cultural period: Basketmaker III (?)
Construction technique: Plain weave and twined
Dimensions: Length 23.5 cm, width 11.5 cm, depth
   0.60 cm
Active elements: Cordage, 2 ply, z-S twist
Average width: 0.15 cm
Passive elements: Cordage, 2 ply, z-S twist
Number of passive units: 26
Number in unit: 1 (except where doubled at toe)
Average width: 0.28 cm
Ties, loops, attachments: Toe: Cordage, 3 ply, s-Z
   twist
Shape: Scalloped toe, heel missing
Start: Scalloped toe start
Body: 2/2 alternate pair twining over doubled warps
   in toe area. Instep to heel woven 4-6 rows of
   1/1 plain weave separated by 1 row of three
   element twining creating a "chain" design
Finish: Missing

Catalog no.: 42SA760 (FS1) 24067
Site: Moqui Canyon Sites, Utah
Collector and date: UCRBASP, 1961
Cultural period: Pueblo II
Construction technique: Plain weave
Dimensions: Length 25.3 cm, width 10.0 cm, depth
   1.3 cm
Active elements: Shredded leaf element
Average width: 0.70 cm
Passive elements: Shredded leaf element, 2 ply, spun
   lightly z and twisted S
Number of passive units: 4
Number in unit: 1
Average width: 1.0 cm
Ties, loops, attachments: Toe: Remnant of tie knotted
   to instep leaf loop which is knotted to a 2 ply
   s-Z twist cordage. Heel: Cordage, heel loop, 2
   ply s-Z twist, looped around warps at each edge.
   Two cords extend from heel loop with one
   broken and the other one knotted to instep
   cordage.
Shape: Right foot shaping, squared toe and heel
Start: At toe one row of twining anchors warps
   that are left with ends frayed and fringed above
   row of twining.
Body: Over-under plain weave for length of sandal.
   Ends frayed on both surfaces
Finish: At heel warps appear split and wrapped
   around adjacent warps with ends protruding.
Other: Structural padding on sole

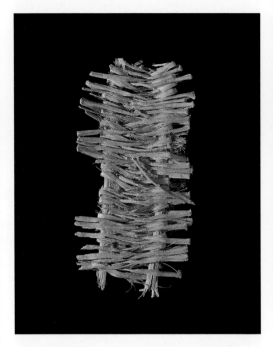 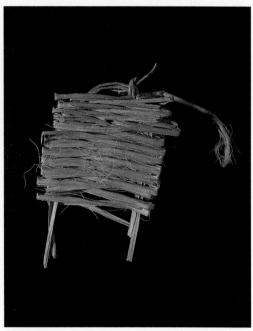

Catalog no.: 42SA643 (FS3.21)
Site: Mosquito Cave, Utah
Collector and date: UCRBASP, 1954
Cultural period: Pueblo II-Pueblo III
Construction technique: Plain weave
Dimensions: Length 18.0 cm, width 9.0 cm, depth 1.10 cm
Active elements: Leaf element unspun, cortex intact
Average width: 0.30 cm
Passive elements: Leaf element unspun, cortex intact
Number of passive units: 2
Number in unit: 2-3?
Average width: 0.96 cm
Ties, loops, attachments: None apparent
Shape: Rounded toe, heel missing
Start: Warps are tied together in one knot at toe.
Body: Over-under plain weave beginning with narrow ends of leaf element on top and ending with shredded wide ends on sole for padding. Wefts encircle warps both tightly and loosely which extends the width of sandal beyond the warp edge.
Finish: Missing
Other: Structural padding on sole

Catalog no.: 2530
Site: Mummy Cave No. 2, Utah
Collector and date: Byron Cummings, University of Utah Expedition, 1914
Cultural period: Unknown
Construction technique: Plain weave
Dimensions: Length 16.0 cm, width 10.0 cm, depth 0.50 cm
Active elements: Leaf element unspun, cortex intact
Average width: 0.45 cm
Passive elements: Leaf element unspun, cortex intact
Number of passive units: 2
Number in unit: 2
Average width: 0.70 cm
Ties, loops, attachments: None apparent
Shape: Rounded toe, heel missing
Start: Warps are tied together at toe in one knot.
Body: Over-under plain weave beginning with narrow ends of leaf element on top and ending with shredded wide ends on sole for padding
Finish: Missing
Other: Structural padding on sole

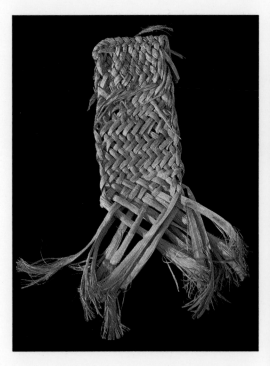
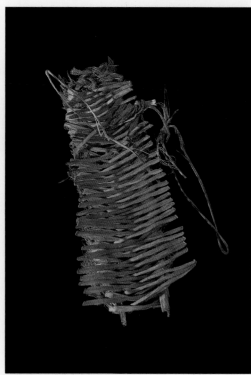

Catalog no.: 2590
Site: Mummy Cave No. 2, Utah
Collector and date: Byron Cummings, University of
 Utah Expedition, 1914
Cultural period: Unknown
Construction technique: Plain weave
Dimensions: Length 21.0 cm, width 9.50 cm, depth
 0.30 cm
Active elements: Leaf element unspun, cortex intact
Average width: 0.47 cm
Passive elements: Leaf element unspun, cortex intact
Number of passive units: 2
Number in unit: 3
Average width: 0.88 cm
Ties, loops, attachments: Heel: Leaf element looped
 around heel area and knotted on upper surface.
 Two additional ties loop through heel loop.
Shape: Rounded toe, heel missing
Start: Missing
Body: Over-under plain weave beginning with
 narrow ends of leaf element on top and ending
 with shredded wide ends on sole for padding
Finish: At heel warps are tied in three knots.
Other: Structural padding on sole

102 Catalog no.: 2563
Site: Mummy Cave No. 2, Utah
Collector and date: Byron Cummings, University of
 Utah Expedition, 1914
Cultural period: Unknown
Construction technique: Plaited
Dimensions: Length 33.0 cm, width 10.0 cm, depth
 1.0 cm
Active elements: Leaf element unspun, cortex intact
Average width: 0.60 cm
Passive elements: N/A
Ties, loops, attachments: None apparent
Shape: Squared toe
Start: Eleven double elements are aligned parallel at
 toe, followed by one row of S twist twining held
 in place by a square knot at one end. The pairs
 of elements are then folded 360° and a 1/1
 interlacement progresses with 2/2 active
 elements for 5 cm at which point the doubling of
 elements end. Ends are left exposed on the
 surface and reverse side.
Body: Twenty-two elements are worked in a 1/1
 plaiting and then shift to a 2/1 transitional row
 followed by a 3/1 plaiting and end with 2/1
 plaiting.
Finish: Unfinished

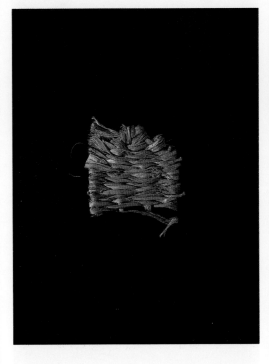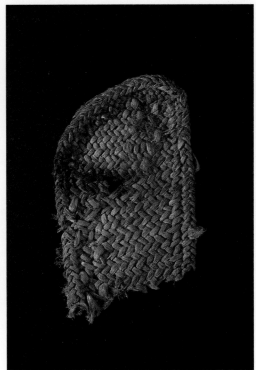

Catalog no.: 2591
Site: Mummy Cave No. 2, Utah
Collector and date: Byron Cummings, University of
  Utah Expedition, 1914
Cultural period: Unknown
Construction technique: Plain weave
Dimensions: Length 6.79 cm, width 7.74 cm, depth
  0.44 cm
Active elements: Leaf element unspun, cortex intact
Average width: 0.34 cm
Passive elements: Leaf element unspun, cortex intact
Number of passive units: 4
Number in unit: 1
Average width: 0.34 cm
Ties, loops, attachments: None apparent
Shape: Rounded toe, heel missing
Start: Warps are tied together at toe in one knot
  which is wrapped with a leaf element.
Body: Over-under plain weave, leaving wide ends
  shredded on sole for padding
Finish: Missing
Other: Structural padding on sole

Catalog no.: 2592
Site: Mummy Cave No. 2, Utah
Collector and date: Byron Cummings, University of
  Utah Expedition, 1914
Cultural period: Unknown
Construction technique: Plaited
Dimensions: Length 18.5 cm, width 11 cm, depth
  0.65 cm
Active elements: Leaf element unspun, cortex intact
Average width: 0.43 cm
Passive elements: N/A
Ties, loops, attachments: None apparent
Shape: Left foot shaping, rounded toe, heel missing
Start: Elements folded at toe for 2/2 plaiting.
  Elements spliced (?) in to create double toe edge
  with shifts of 2/1/2 to facilitate shaping. Elements
  pulled in at edges with every other element
  shifting to over three creating a herringbone
  selvage. Exhausted wide ends left frayed on toe
Other: Structural padding on sole. Charred

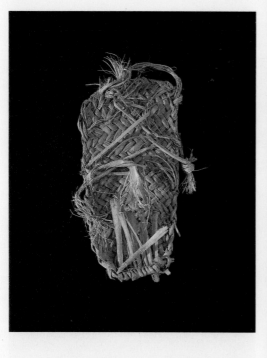

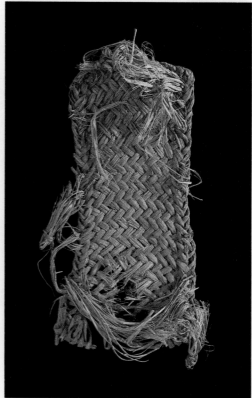

Catalog no.: 2596
Site: Mummy Cave No. 2, Utah
Collector and date: Byron Cummings, University of
Utah Expedition, 1914
Cultural period: Unknown
Construction technique: Plaited
Dimensions: Length 17.0 cm, width 9.0 cm, depth
1.0 cm
Active elements: Leaf element unspun, cortex intact
Average width: 0.54 cm
Passive elements: N/A
Ties, loops, attachments: Toe: Two leaf element ties
loop and stitch into edges. A center tie catches
these loops and laces together in middle of
sandal. Edge: Ties at edge and tie remnants near
heel
Shape: Left foot shaping, rounded toe and heel
Start: 28 elements are aligned parallel and twined,
then folded with short ends at toe so twining
shows on only one surface.
Body: 2/2 plaiting for forward one-third of sandal.
Shift of 2/3/1/2 drops one element, which draws
sandal in for shaping. One more element is
dropped near heel.
Finish: Left element forms a bar across heel. One
half of the remaining elements wrap around bar
and extend on top of sandal. Remaining elements
are cut short on sole.

Catalog no.: 2597
Site: Mummy Cave No. 2, Utah
Collector and date: Byron Cummings, University of
Utah Expedition, 1914
Cultural period: Unknown
Construction technique: Plaited
Dimensions: Length 26.0 cm, width 11.0 cm, depth
0.97 cm
Active elements: Leaf element unspun, cortex intact
Average width: 0.55 cm
Passive elements: N/A
Ties, loops, attachments: Toe: Leaf element knotted
at one toe edge and looped through center of
toe, ending on opposite toe edge. Heel: Leaf
element looped through edge ties and knotted.
Edge: leaf elements looped and stitched into
sandal along both edges
Shape: Slightly rounded toe, heel missing
Start: 24(?) elements are doubled at toe only and
plaited double for a short distance. One row of
single twining near toe
Body: 2/2 twill plaiting for length of sandal. Two
elements are dropped from each edge near ball
of foot for shaping.
Finish: Missing

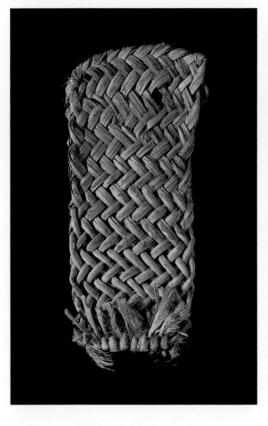
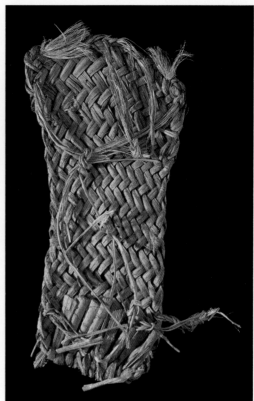

Catalog no.: 2598
Site: Mummy Cave No. 2, Utah
Collector and date: Byron Cummings, University of
   Utah Expedition, 1914
Cultural period: Unknown
Construction technique: Plaited
Dimensions: Length 23.1 cm, width 10.5 cm, depth
   0.64 cm
Active elements: Leaf element unspun, cortex intact
Average width: 0.73 cm
Passive elements: N/A
Ties, loops, attachments: None apparent
Shape: Left foot shaping, slightly rounded toe and
   squared heel
Start: Ten elements are folded double at toe.
   Before folding one row of twining binds
   elements. After folding twining only evident on
   one side
Body: 2/2 twill plaiting using doubled elements for
   approximately one-third of sandal. Doubled
   elements are then dropped and 2/2 plaiting
   continues to heel using single elements.
Finish: At heel one edge element forms a transverse
   bar where every other element folds over and
   protrudes on upper surface. Odd elements are
   left protruding on sole.

Catalog no.: 2600
Site: Mummy Cave No. 2, Utah
Collector and date: Byron Cummings, University of
   Utah Expedition, 1914
Cultural period: Unknown
Construction technique: Plaited
Dimensions: Length 26.0 cm, width 13.0 cm (toe),
   depth 0.50 cm
Active elements: Leaf element, unspun, cortex intact
Average width: 0.59 cm
Passive elements: N/A
Ties, loops, attachments: Toe: Loop of leaf element
   with square knot at top of loop. A second loop
   consists of two yucca leaves knotted on top of
   instep and extending from edge to edge at base
   of toes. Ends are long and possibly connected to
   heel loop. Heel: Loops of two leaves are secured
   at each edge by stitching into sandal.
Shape: Right foot shaping, slightly rounded toe and
   heel
Start: Elements doubled at toe
Body: 2/2 twill plaiting using doubled elements until
   exhausted, at which point plaiting continues with
   single elements. Several elements dropped in
   body for shaping. Weaving pulled tighter at
   instep to heel of sandal
Finish: At heel one active element from left side
   forms a bar across heel. Every other element is
   wrapped around bar to upper side of sandal.
   Other elements truncated on sole
Other: Two horizontal leaf elements were woven
   across sandal.

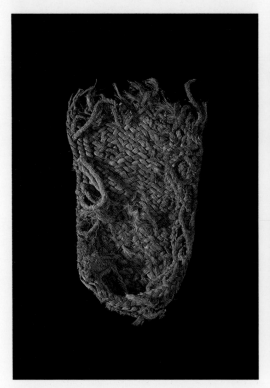
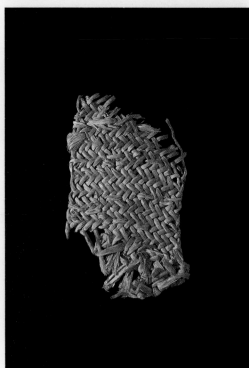

Catalog no.: 2602
Site: Mummy Cave No. 2, Utah
Collector and date: Byron Cummings, University of Utah Expedition, 1914
Cultural period: Unknown
Construction technique: Plaited
Dimensions: Length 16.5 cm, width 11.0 cm, depth 0.44 cm
Active elements: Leaf element unspun, cortex intact
Average width: 0.36 cm
Passive elements: N/A
Ties, loops, attachments: Edge: Cordage 2 ply, s-Z twist is stitched along both edges. Two loops from each edge tuck under heel.
Shape: Toe missing, round cupped heel
Start: Missing
Body: 2/2 twill plaiting with edges pulled tightly to create a rolled triple border. Shifts may be 2/1/2 near heel. Exhausted wide ends left frayed on sole
Finish: At heel ends appear protruding on outer heel.
Other: Structural padding on sole

Catalog no.: 2604
Site: Mummy Cave No. 2, Utah
Collector and date: Byron Cummings, University of Utah Expedition, 1914
Cultural period: Unknown
Construction technique: Plaited
Dimensions: Length 16.0 cm, width 10.0 cm, depth 1.0 cm
Active elements: Leaf element unspun, cortex intact
Average width: 0.37 cm
Passive elements: N/A
Ties, loops, attachments: None apparent
Shape: Fragmentary
Start: Disarticulated
Body: 2/2 diagonal twill plaiting, single elements
Finish: Some disarticulation. Remaining elements are alternately folded back on top and bottom, tucked under transverse elements, then clipped.
Other: At regular intervals supplemental leaf elements are woven horizontally in a running stitch.

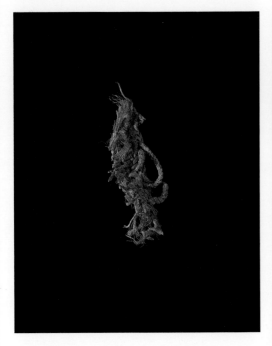

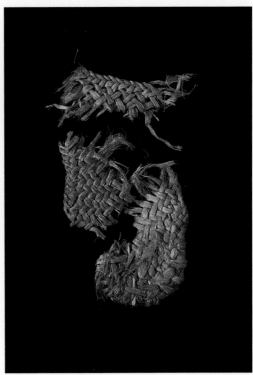

Catalog no.: 2605
Site: Mummy Cave No. 2, Utah
Collector and date: Byron Cummings, University of
  Utah Expedition, 1914
Cultural period: Unknown
Construction technique: Plaited
Dimensions: Overall of three fragments together:
  Length 21.0 cm, width 9.0 cm, depth 0.40 cm.
Active elements: Leaf element unspun, cortex intact
Average width: 0.50 cm
Passive elements: N/A
Ties, loops, attachments: Toe: Cordage element 3 ply,
  z-S twist
Shape: Rounded toe, heel missing
Start: Elements appear folded at toe
Body: 2/2 plaiting with shifts of 2/3/2 and 2/1/1/2
Finish: Missing
Other: Structural padding on sole

Catalog no.: AR3931 92.1
Site: Mummy Cave No. 2, Utah
Collector and date: Byron Cummings, University of
  Utah Expedition, 1914
Cultural period: Unknown
Construction technique: Plaited
Dimensions: Length 14.0 cm, width 3.50 cm, depth
  1.0 cm
Active elements: Leaf element unspun, cortex intact
Average width: 0.24 cm
Passive elements: N/A
Ties, loops, attachments: Edge: Cordage 2 ply, s-Z
  twist, loops along edge stitching into body of
  sandal
Shape: Unknown, fragmentary
Start and Finish: Missing
Body: 2/2 twill plaiting with edge pulled tightly

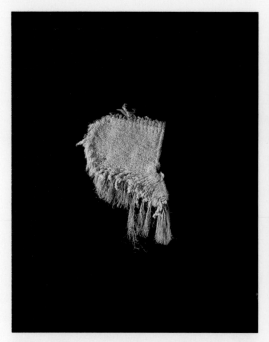

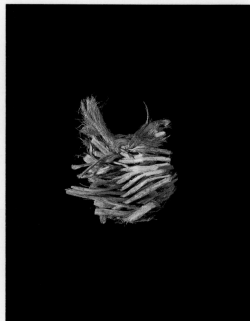

108 *Catalog no.:* 2818
Site: Navajo John Cave, Arizona
Collector and date: Byron Cummings, University of
  Utah Expedition, 1909
Cultural period: Basketmaker III(?)
Construction technique: Twined
Dimensions: Length 10.5 cm, width 6.5 cm, depth
  0.65 cm
Active elements: Cordage, 2 ply, z-S twist
Average width: 0.14 cm
Passive elements: Cordage, 2 ply, z-S twist
Number of passive units: 19(?)
Number in unit: 1 (except where doubled at heel)
Average width: 0.19 cm
Ties, loops, attachments: None apparent
Shape: Unknown, fragmentary
Start and Finish: Missing
Body: 2/2 alternate pair twining on most of
  fragment over doubled warps. Plain twining near
  short exposed warp ends where doubled
  elements have been dropped
Other: Near end of fragment the wefts of the plain
  twining appear dyed yellow or gold

Catalog no.: 2256
Site: Pine Tree House, Arizona
Collector and date: Byron Cummings, University of
  Utah Expedition, 1914
Cultural period: Unknown
Construction technique: Plain weave
Dimensions: Length 7.0 cm, width 8.2 cm, depth
  2.25 cm
Active elements: Leaf element unspun, cortex intact
Average width: 0.58 cm
Passive elements: Leaf element unspun, cortex intact
Number of passive units: 2
Number in unit: 2(?)
Average width: 0.66 cm
Ties, loops, attachments: None apparent
Shape: Fragmentary
Start: Unknown
Body: Over-under plain weave beginning with
  narrow ends of leaf element on top and ending
  with shredded wide ends on sole for padding.
  Short wefts encircle warps tightly but ends
  extend beyond sandal edge.
Finish: At heel(?) warps are tied in two knots.
Other: Structural padding on sole

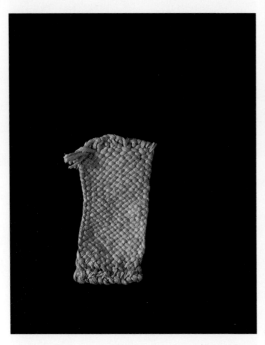

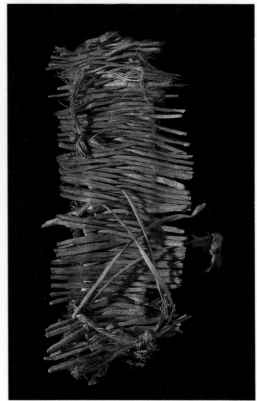

Catalog no.: 2257
Site: Pine Tree House, Arizona
Collector and date: Byron Cummings, University of
    Utah Expedition, 1914
Cultural period: Unknown
Construction technique: Plaited
Dimensions: Length 11.2 cm, width 6.0 cm, depth
    0.40 cm
Active elements: Leaf element unspun, cortex intact
Average width: 0.32 cm
Passive elements: N/A
Ties, loops, attachments: None apparent
Shape: Right foot shaping, rounded toe and squared
    heel
Start: Twelve elements are folded at toe so one
    end is long and the other is short. On left side
    short ends are plaited for one or two intervals
    then left protruding on sole. On right side short
    elements wrap over a transverse element and
    protrude on sole.
Body: 1/1 plaiting for length of sandal drawing in
    tighter at middle.
Finish: At heel elements are secured with one row
    of twining. Ends folded back toward upper side
    and clipped short

Catalog no.: 2531
Site: Pine Tree House, Arizona
Collector and date: Byron Cummings, University of
    Utah Expedition, 1914
Cultural period: Unknown
Construction technique: Plain weave
Dimensions: Length 25.5 cm, width 10.5 cm, depth
    1.4 cm
Active elements: Leaf element unspun, cortex intact
Average width: 0.34 cm
Passive elements: Leaf element unspun, cortex intact
Number of passive units: 2
Number in unit: 2(?)
Average width: 0.58 cm
Ties, loops, attachments: Toe: Broken toe loop, Z
    twisted leaf element with one knot. Heel: Loop,
    S twisted leaf element with one knot. Two single
    leaf element attachments, cortex intact, one with
    a knot, extending toward toe loop
Shape: Rounded toe and heel
Start: Warps are tied together at toe in one knot.
Body: Over-under plain weave with narrow ends of
    leaf element on top and ending with shredded
    wide ends on sole for padding. Short wefts
    encircle warps tightly but ends extend beyond
    sandal edge.
Finish: Warps tied together at heel with two knots
Other: Structural padding on sole

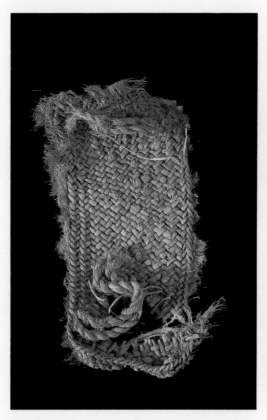
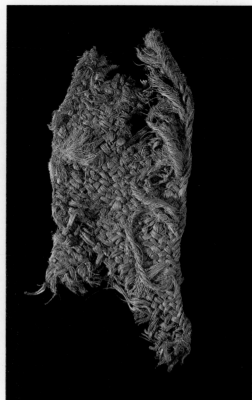

110

Catalog no.: 2601
Site: Pine Tree House, Arizona
Collector and date: Byron Cummings, University of
Utah Expedition, 1914
Cultural period: Unknown
Construction technique: Plaited
Dimensions: Length 23.5 cm, width 11.0 cm, depth
1.82 cm
Active elements: Leaf element unspun, cortex intact
Average width: 0.46 cm
Passive elements: N/A
Ties, loops, attachments: Toe: Cordage 2 ply, s-Z
twist loops at toe and tied with a leaf element.
Heel: Cordage 2 ply, s-Z twist loop attached to
sandal at left side. Leaf element near heel is
doubled and knotted on sole.
Shape: Right foot shaping, rounded toe with toe jog
and cupped heel
Start: Ten(?) elements folded at toe to form 20
active elements. One more element folded for
toe jog
Body: 2/2 twill plaiting for length of sandal with
wide ends of leaf element left shredded on sole
for padding. Edges plaited tightly to give a raised
effect. Heel also plaited tightly to create a
cupped heel
Finish: At heel elements are knotted twice so all
ends protrude down toward sole.
Other: Structural padding on sole. Stitching on
upper side with ends shredded on sole

Catalog no.: 2254
Site: Priestess Cave, Arizona
Collector and date: Byron Cummings, University of
Utah Expedition, 1914
Cultural period: Unknown
Construction technique: Plaited
Dimensions: Length 26.0 cm, width 12.0 cm, depth
1.5 cm
Active elements: Leaf element unspun, cortex intact
Average width: 0.47 cm
Passive elements: N/A
Ties, loops, attachments: Edge: Cordage 2 ply, s-Z
twist and leaf element twisted S are evident
along stable edge and are anchored with
overhand knots on sole. Elements are looped
along edge. Remnants of loops on opposite edge.
Shape: Unknown
Start and Finish: Missing
Body: 2/2 twill plaiting with irregular shifts including
a 2/3/2 at edges
Other: Possible vertical stitching

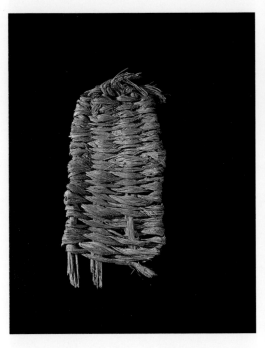
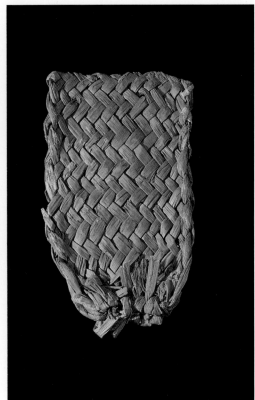

Catalog no.: 2255
Site: Priestess Cave, Arizona
Collector and date: Byron Cummings, University of
  Utah Expedition, 1914
Cultural period: Unknown
Construction technique: Plain weave
Dimensions: Length 16.0 cm, width 8.0 cm, depth
  1.83 cm
Active elements: Leaf elements unspun, cortex intact
Average width: 0.51 cm
Passive elements: Leaf element unspun, cortex intact
Number of passive units: 4
Number in unit: 2
Average width: 0.70 cm
Ties, loops, attachments: Three pieces of leaf
  element pierce sandal with only stubs remaining.
Shape: Completed end round
Start or Finish: Four doubled elements are crossed
  over one another and knotted with half-hitch
  knots.
Body: Over-under plain weave for length of sandal

Catalog no.: 2499
Site: Priestess Cave, Arizona
Collector and date: Byron Cummings, University of
  Utah Expedition, 1914
Cultural period: Unknown
Construction technique: Plaited
Dimensions: Length 20.5 cm, width 12.0 cm, depth
  0.5 cm
Active elements: Leaf element unspun, cortex intact
Average width: 0.78 cm
Passive elements: N/A
Ties, loops, attachments: None apparent
Shape: Squared toe and rounded heel
Start: Eleven single elements folded at toe to form
  22 elements
Body: 2/2 twill plaiting for length of sandal
Finish: Ends are alternately folded back on top and
  bottom, tucked under transverse elements, then
  clipped.

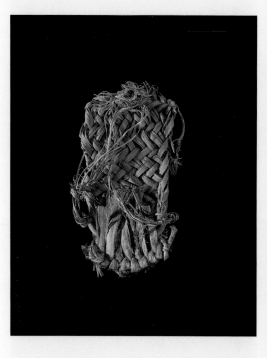

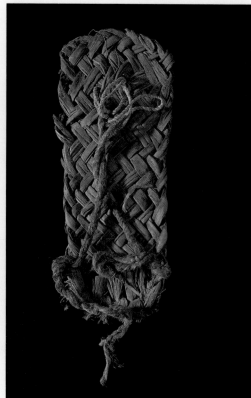

Catalog no.: 2500
Site: Priestess Cave, Arizona
Collector and date: Byron Cummings, University of
Utah Expedition, 1914
Cultural period: Unknown
Construction technique: Plaited
Dimensions: Length 15.0 cm, width 8.0 cm, depth
0.90 cm
Active elements: Leaf element unspun, cortex intact
Average width: 0.54 cm
Passive elements: N/A
Ties, loops, attachments: Toe and Edge: A leaf
element is inserted into each toe edge of sandal
from the upper surface. Ends are frayed to
anchor. Elements emerge on upper surface again,
cross each other, and attach on opposite edge
with twisting and a knot.
Shape: Rounded toe and squared heel
Start: Ten elements are aligned parallel and twined
with one row of S twining. Elements are then
folded to make 20 active elements. Because of
fold twining is visible on only one surface.
Body: 2/2 twill plaiting with shift of 2/3/1/2 at
selvages which are pulled in. Shift of 2/3/2 near
heel where two elements have been eliminated
for shaping
Finish: At heel half of the elements are ended on
sole. The remaining elements knot over a
transverse bar that is anchored at each edge.
Ends protrude on upper surface.
Other: Structural padding on sole

Catalog no.: 2501
Site: Priestess Cave, Arizona
Collector and date: Byron Cummings, University of
Utah Expedition, 1914
Cultural period: Unknown
Construction technique: Plaited
Dimensions: Length 23.5 cm, width 9.2 cm, depth
0.70 cm
Active elements: Leaf element, unspun, cortex intact
Average width: 0.74 cm
Passive elements: N/A
Ties, loops, attachments: Toe: Two loops of 2 ply, s-Z
twist cordage are stitched through sandal four
times. Heel: Cordage 2 ply, s-Z twist looped
around toe cord and extended to instep then to
heel where cord is stitched, twisted around itself
twice, and stitched through side edge of heel and
knotted with other end of heel loop
Shape: Squared toe and rounded heel
Start: Active elements doubled at toe
Body: 2/2 twill plaiting for length of sandal
Finish: At heel five ends are folded under an
additional element, then brought to top of sandal
and left protruding. Other ends are folded over
additional element and woven back in to create
a two-layer finish.

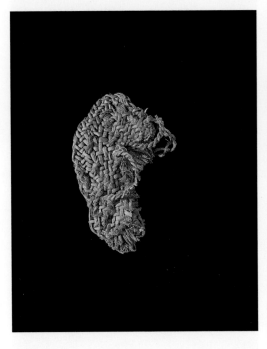

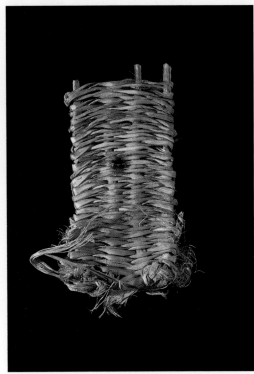

Catalog no.: 2580
Site: Priestess Cave, Arizona
Collector and date: Byron Cummings, University of
 Utah Expedition, 1914
Cultural period: Unknown
Construction technique: Plaited
Dimensions: Length 13.0 cm, width 7.0 cm, depth
 1.064 cm
Active elements: Leaf element unspun, cortex intact
Average width: 0.31 cm
Passive elements: N/A
Ties, loops, attachments: Two complete cordage
 loops 2 ply, z-S twist extend from center to
 edge. One remnant tie at edge
Shape: Curved finished edge, fragmentary piece
Start: Folded starts on both layers
Body: 2/2 twill plaiting with 3/2 and 2/1 shifts for
 shaping
Finish: Missing
Other: Two fragments sewn together with cordage
 2 ply, s-Z twist

Catalog no.: 2581
Site: Priestess Cave, Arizona
Collector and date: Byron Cummings, University of
 Utah Expedition, 1914
Cultural period: Unknown
Construction technique: Plain weave
Dimensions: Length 18.9 cm, width 8.25 cm, depth
 1.0 cm
Active elements: Leaf element unspun, cortex intact
Average width: 0.38 cm
Passive elements: Leaf element unspun, cortex intact
Number of passive units: 4
Number in unit: 2
Average width: 0.60 cm
Ties, loops, attachments: Heel: At each side a lightly
 twisted leaf element is inserted through a turn in
 the weft and then twisted back on itself.
Shape: Unknown
Start or Finish: Two knots remaining where warps
 are brought together
Body: Over-under plain weave for length of piece
Other: Structural padding on sole

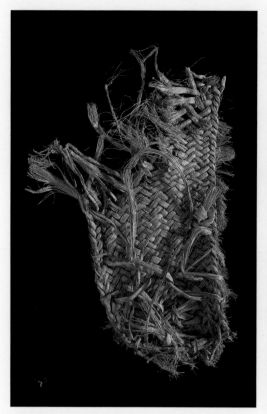
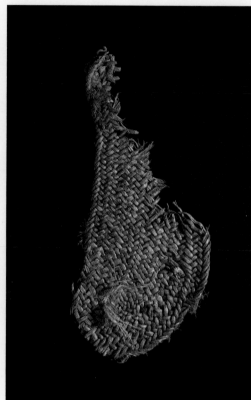

114   *Catalog no.:* 2582
Site: Priestess Cave, Arizona
Collector and date: Byron Cummings, University of
   Utah Expedition, 1914
Cultural period: Unknown
Construction technique: Plaited
Dimensions: Length 23.5 cm, width 11.0 cm, depth
   0.50 cm
Active elements: Leaf element unspun, cortex intact
Average width: 0.48 cm
Passive elements: N/A
Ties, loops, attachments: Toe: Leaf element loop and
   tie that attach to lacing. Edge: Leaf element loops
   and stitches into body of sandal at both edges.
   Loops connected with lacing
Shape: Right foot shaping, rounded toe area, heel
   missing
Start and Finish: Missing
Body: 2/2 twill plaiting for body of sandal. Exhausted
   ends left frayed on sole
Other: Structural padding on sole

Catalog no.: 2583
Site: Priestess Cave, Arizona
Collector and date: Byron Cummings, University of
   Utah Expedition, 1914
Cultural period: Unknown
Construction technique: Plaited
Dimensions: Length 25.0 cm, width 10.5 cm, depth
   0.70 cm
Active elements: Leaf element unspun, cortex intact
Average width: 0.36 cm
Passive elements: N/A
Ties, loops, attachments: Toe: Fragmented toe loop.
   Heel: Knot evident on sole
Shape: Left foot shaping, round tapered toe with
   toe jog, heel missing
Start: Active elements appear folded at toe with a
   folded element added at toe jog.
Body: 2/2 twill plaiting with 2/1/2 shifts for rounding
   of toe and a shift of 2/3/2 at edges. Exhausted
   ends left frayed on sole
Finish: Missing
Other: Structural padding on sole

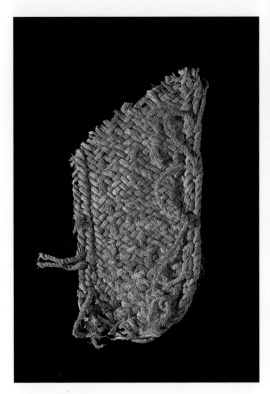

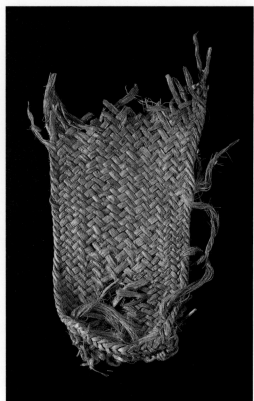

Catalog no.: 2586
Site: Priestess Cave, Utah
Collector and date: Byron Cummings, University of
    Utah Expedition, 1914
Cultural period: Unknown
Construction technique: Plaited
Dimensions: Length 21.0 cm, width 10.5 cm, depth
    0.63 cm
Active elements: Leaf element unspun, cortex intact
Average width: 0.47 cm
Passive elements: N/A
Ties, loops, attachments: Heel: Cordage 2 ply, s-Z
    twist. Edge: Cordage loops 2 ply, s-Z twist
Shape: Left foot shaping, rounded heel, toe missing
Start: Missing, but elements appear folded.
Body: 2/2 twill plaiting for length of sandal, with
    shift of 2/3/2 at selvages which are pulled tight
    to create two ridges on each side. Exhausted
    weft ends frayed on sole
Finish: End finish missing
Other: Broad horizontal and vertical stitches of 2
    ply, s-Z twist cordage appear to be structural
    and make a knot in between stitches on sole.
    Structural padding on sole

Catalog no.: AR1943 87.1
Site: Priestess Cave, Utah
Collector and date: Byron Cummings, University of
    Utah Expedition, 1914
Cultural period: Unknown
Construction technique: Plaited
Dimensions: Length 26.0 cm, width 13.0 cm, depth
    0.53 cm
Active elements: Leaf element unspun, cortex intact
Average width: 0.48 cm
Passive elements: N/A
Ties, loops, attachments: Edge: Separated leaf
    element twisted S is looped into body of sandal
    at right edge. Heel: Two S twisted separated leaf
    elements knotted at both sides of heel from
    inside
Shape: Left(?) foot shaping, cupped heel, toe
    missing
Start: Missing
Body: 2/2 twill plaiting for length of sandal. 2/3/3
    shift at side selvages and heel. Heel is drawn in
    tight.
Finish: At heel ends appear looped around adjacent
    elements and clipped short.

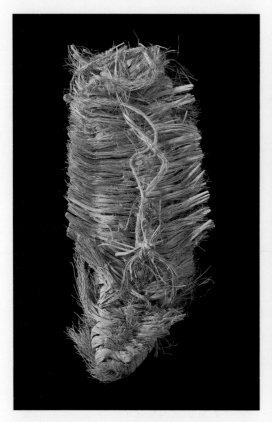 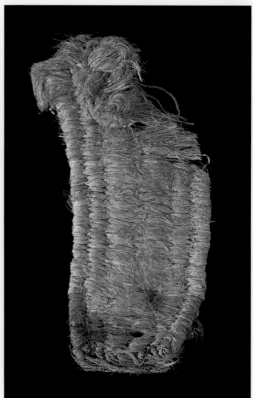

116   *Catalog no.:* 42SA681 (FS4.2) 24070
Site: Rehab Center, Utah
Collector and date: UCRBASP 1961
Cultural period: Pueblo II
Construction technique: Plain weave
Dimensions: Length 25.5 cm, width 11.5 cm, depth 2.4 cm
Active elements: Leaf element unspun, cortex intact
Average width: 0.5 cm
Passive elements: Leaf element unspun, cortex intact
Number of passive units: 2
Number in unit: 1
Average width: 1.37 cm
Ties, loops, attachments: Heel and Toe: Remnants of leaf element attachments twisted S
Shape: Rounded toe and heel
Start: Warps are tied together at toe in one knot.
Body: Over-under plain weave beginning with narrow ends of leaf element on top and ending with shredded wide ends on sole for padding. Wefts encircle warps tightly. Ends extend beyond warp edge of sandal.
Finish: Warps are tied at heel in one knot.
Other: Structural padding on sole

Catalog no.: 42SA681 (FS28.1) 24070
Site: Rehab Center, Utah
Collector and date: UCRBASP, 1961
Cultural period: Pueblo II
Construction technique: Plain weave
Dimensions: Length 28.5 cm, width 11.5 cm, depth 1.50 cm
Active elements: Shredded leaf element, twisted S and Z
Average width: 0.55 cm
Passive elements: Separated leaf element unspun, cortex intact, two groups twisted together S
Number of passive units: 6
Number in unit: 1
Average width: 1.19 cm
Ties, loops, attachments: Toe: Cordage, tie, 2 ply, Z twist (each ply 2 ply, twisted S with each ply 2 ply, s-Z twist). Loop of fine 2 ply s-Z twist cordage around middle warp. Cordage appears dyed with red ocher.
Shape: Squared toe and heel
Start: Twining appears to have held warps secure with warps left fringed at toe. Also evidence of warp knots
Body: Over-under plain weave for length of sandal. Shredded yucca weft has been gathered together for appropriate width of weft and twisted as it is woven. This gives an "S" twist in one direction and a "Z" twist in the opposite direction. Ends left frayed on sole
Finish: Warp ends knotted several times on adjacent warps
Other: Structural padding on sole.

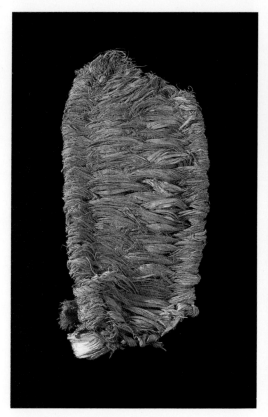

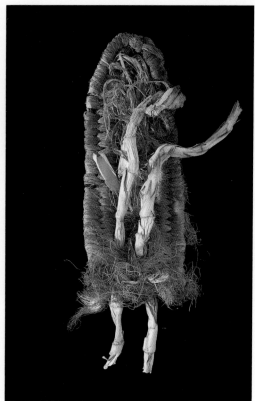

Catalog no.: 42SA681 (FS76.14) 24070
Site: Rehab Center, Utah
Collector and date: UCRBASP 1961
Cultural period: Pueblo II
Construction technique: Plain weave
Dimensions: Length 23 cm, width 11.5 cm, depth
   1.04 cm
Active elements: Shredded leaf element unspun,
   cortex intact, twisted S and Z
Average width: 0.75 cm
Passive elements: Leaf element unspun, cortex intact
Number of passive units: 4
Number in unit: 1
Average width: 0.63 cm
Ties, loops, attachments: Remnant of one tie looped
   around warp and knotted
Shape: Right foot shaping, rounded heel, toe
   missing
Start: Missing
Body: Tightly packed plain weave continues to heel.
   Shredded yucca weft has been gathered together
   for appropriate width of weft and twisted as it is
   woven. This gives an "S" twist in one direction
   and a "Z" twist in the opposite direction. Weft
   ends form padding on sole.
Finish: Warp ends at heel are successively wrapped
   around the next warp and the end tucked into
   the body, across the heel.
Other: Structural padding

Catalog no.: 42SA681 (FS103.24) 24070
Site: Rehab Center, Utah
Collector and date: UCRBASP 1961
Cultural period: Pueblo II
Construction technique: Plain weave
Dimensions: Length 21.3 cm, width 8.3 cm, depth
   1.60 cm
Active elements: Leaf element unspun, cortex intact
Average width: 0.58 cm
Passive elements: Leaf element unspun, cortex intact
Number of passive units: 6
Number in unit: 1
Average width: 0.48 cm
Ties, loops, attachments: Toe: Leaf element looped
   through sandal in middle of toe. Another tie
   forms loop at instep knotting to toe loop. Heel:
   Loop of leaf element knotted to tie at right side
   that extends to instep loop
Shape: Squared toe and round cupped heel
Start: Three warps are folded at toe to form six
   warps.
Body: Over-under plain weave for length of sandal
Finish: At heel outer warps are knotted together
   tightly to form cupped heel. Second and fifth
   warps knot as do the middle two warps.
Other: Structural padding on sole. Two stalks of
   Zeamays leaf have been pierced through toe
   areas of sandal and protrude on sole, serving no
   apparent structural purpose.

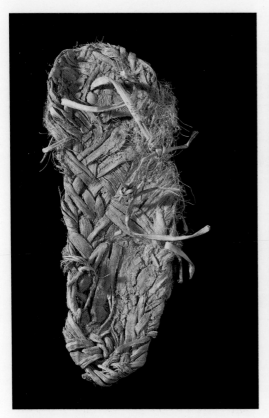

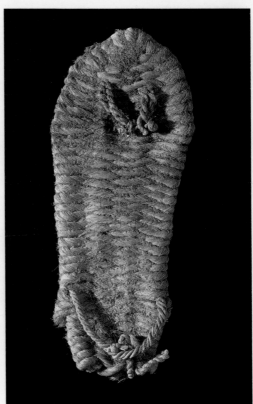

Catalog no.: 42WS4 13608
Site: Santa Barbara Creek, Veyo, Utah
Collector and date: Statewide Survey, 1949
Cultural period: Unknown
Construction technique: Plain weave
Dimensions: Length 29 cm, width 12 cm, depth 1.5
    cm
Active elements: Shredded leaf element, twisted S
    and Z
Average width: 0.66 cm
Passive elements: Cordage, 2 ply, s-Z twist
Number of passive units: 4
Number in unit: 1
Average width: 0.4 cm
Ties, loops, attachments: Toe: Two 2-ply z-S twist
    cordage loops side by side centered in toe.
    Knotted cordage attached to toe loops. Heel:
    Cordage, loop 4 ply, z-S twist with looped knot
    in center of loop. Other heel cordage: 2 ply, s-Z
    twist
Shape: Left foot shaping, rounded toe with slight
    point and squared heel
Start: Two cordage warps folded at toe (one inside
    the other) to form four warps
Body: Tightly packed plain weave continues to heel.
    Shredded yucca weft has been gathered together
    for appropriate width of weft and twisted as it is
    woven. This gives an "S" twist in one direction
    and a "Z" twist in the opposite direction.
Finish: At heel, 2 warp cords cross each other,
    tucking into opposite channel. It appears one
    cordage at heel has been inserted where these
    warp cords cross.

// \\\ /// \\\ /// \\\ /// \\\ /// \\\ /// \\\ /// \\\ ///

118   Catalog no.: 42SA15 23753
       Site: San Juan County, Utah
       Collector and date: Statewide Archaeological Survey,
           1952-53
       Cultural period: Unknown
       Construction technique: Plaited
       Dimensions: Length 27.0 cm, width 9.5 cm, depth
           1.56 cm
       Active elements: Leaf element unspun, cortex intact
       Average width: 0.80 cm
       Passive elements: N/A
       Ties, loops, attachments: Toe: Leaf element loop
           stitched across toe and protrudes to surface at
           toe center and extends to instep which is
           knotted to broken leaf elements.Edge: One
           remnant on each side
       Shape: Right foot shaping, rounded toe and heel
       Start: Active elements folded at toe.
       Body: Twill plaiting with irregular pattern and shifts.
       Finish: Elements gathered tighter at heel and woven
           back to the surface of sandal.

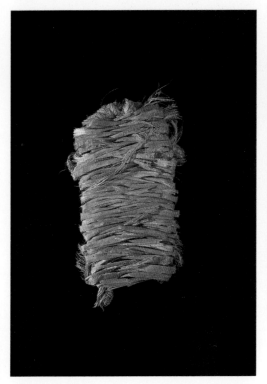

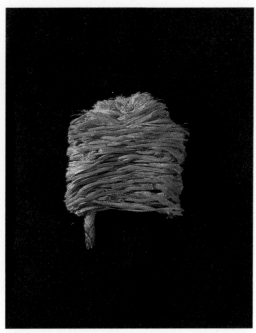

Catalog no.: 644
Site: Sega at Sosa (Tsegi Hatsosie) Canyon, Arizona
Collector and date: Byron Cummings, University of
Utah Expedition, 1909
Cultural period: Unknown
Construction technique: Plain weave
Dimensions: Length 14.0 cm, width 8.0 cm, depth
1.0 cm
Active elements: Leaf element unspun, cortex intact
Average width: 0.44 cm
Passive elements: Braid, three strand, leaf elements
unspun, cortex intact
Number of passive units: 2
Number in unit: 1
Average width: 0.56 cm
Ties, loops, attachments: Toe: Two remnant ties of
leaf elements on sole
Shape: Rounded toe
Start: Warp braid folded at toe and wrapped with
weft
Body: Over-under plain weave, beginning with
narrow ends on top near center of sandal and
ending with shredded wide ends on sole for
padding
Finish: Unknown
Other: Structural padding on sole

Catalog no.: 645
Site: Sega at Sosa (Tsegi Hatsosie) Canyon, Arizona
Collector and date: Byron Cummings, University of
Utah Expedition, 1909
Cultural period: Unknown
Construction technique: Plain weave
Dimensions: Length 12.0 cm, width 10.0 cm, depth
1.50 cm
Active elements: Leaf element unspun, cortex intact
Average width: 0.39 cm
Passive elements: Braid, three-strand leaf element,
unspun, cortex intact
Number of passive units: 2
Number in unit: 1
Average width: 0.78 cm
Ties, loops, attachments: Edge: Stubs on both sides
near toe
Shape: Rounded toe
Start: Warps are knotted together at toe and
wrapped with weft.
Body: Over-under plain weave beginning with
narrow leaves on top near center. Wide ends
shredded on sole for padding
Finish: Unknown
Other: Structural padding on sole

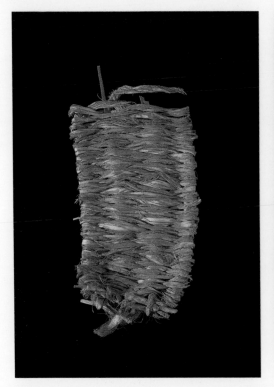
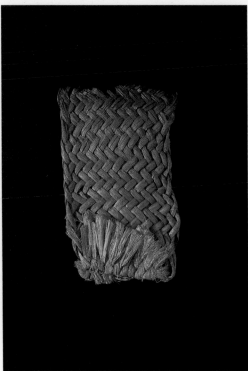

120 *Catalog no.:* 646
Site: Sega at Sosa (Tsegi Hatsosie) Canyon, Arizona
Collector and date: Byron Cummings, University of
    Utah Expedition, 1909
Cultural period: Unknown
Construction technique: Plain weave
Dimensions: Length 14.67 cm, width 9.47 cm, depth
    0.69 cm
Active elements: Leaf element unspun, cortex intact
Average width: 0.56 cm
Passive elements: Leaf element unspun, cortex intact
Number of passive units: 4
Number in unit: 2
Average width: 0.47 cm
Ties, loops, attachments: None apparent
Shape: Squared heel, toe missing
Start: Unknown
Body: Over-under plain weave for length of sandal
    with ends left frayed on sole
Finish: At heel warps are tied in four knots.
Other: Structural padding on sole

Catalog no.: 647
Site: Sega at Sosa (Tsegi Hatsosie) Canyon, Arizona
Collector and date: Byron Cummings, University of
    Utah Expedition, 1909
Cultural period: Unknown
Construction technique: Plaited
Dimensions: Length 15.1 cm, width 8.7 cm, depth
    0.47 cm
Active elements: Leaf element unspun, cortex intact
Average width: 0.53 cm
Passive elements: N/A
Ties, loops, attachments: None apparent
Shape: Toe missing, squared heel
Start: Missing
Body: 2/2 twill plaiting with shifts of 2/1/1/2 and a
    single row of 1/1 where sandal expands slightly
    at ball of foot
Finish: At heel every other end is looped over a
    transverse bar onto upper surface of sandal.
    Alternate ends are truncated on sole.
Other: Toe end charred

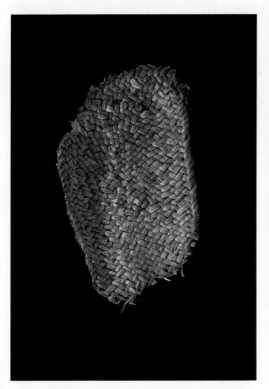

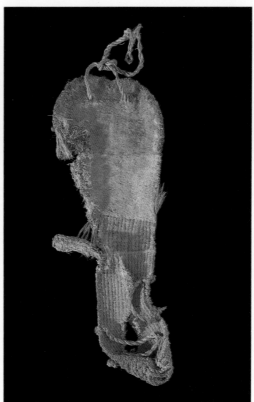

Catalog no.: 648
Site: Sega at Sosa (Tsegi Hatsosie) Canyon, Arizona
Collector and date: Byron Cummings, University of
   Utah Expedition, 1909
Cultural period: Unknown
Construction technique: Plaited
Dimensions: Length 17.5 cm, width 10.6 cm, depth
   0.73 cm
Active elements: Leaf element unspun, cortex intact
Average width: 0.32 cm
Passive elements: N/A
Ties, loops, attachments: Toe and Edge: Remnants of
   knots on sole
Shape: Left foot shaping, tapered toe, heel missing
Start: Active elements folded at toe
Body: 2/2 twill plaiting with three shifts of 2/3/1/2 in
   toe area. Two elements are dropped at
   midsection. Edges are pulled tightly.
Finish: Missing

Catalog no.: 691
Site: Sega at Sosa (Tsegi Hatsosie) Canyon, Arizona
Collector and date: Byron Cummings, University of
   Utah Expedition, 1909
Cultural period: Basketmaker III
Construction technique: Composite
Dimensions: Length 26.0 cm, width 9.6 cm, depth
   0.66 cm
Active elements: Cordage, 2 ply, z-S twist
Average width: 0.11 cm
Passive elements: Cordage, 3 ply, z-S twist
Number of passive units: 27-28
Number in unit: 1 (except where doubled at toe)
Average width: 0.12 cm
Ties, loops, attachments: Toe: cordage, loop 3 ply,
   s-Z twist, knotted at toe. Heel: cordage, 2 ply,
   z-S twist, on right side from heel. Edge: Near
   heel 2 ply cordage looped into both sides of
   sandal and knotted, z-S twist.
Shape: Scalloped toe and puckered heel
Start: Scalloped toe start
Body: 2/2 alternate pair twining over doubled warps
   for forward one-third section of sandal at which
   point doubled warps end. Half of forward
   section appears dyed with yellow and/or red.
   Middle section is a geometric pattern in burnt
   orange, yellow, brown(?), and natural. Geometric
   design possible using A & B weaving. Weaving as
   pattern is not clear on reverse side. Remaining
   length of sandal woven in raised geometric
   pattern
Finish: Puckered heel finish. Several warps form heel
   cord. Remaining ends tuck inside of sandal.

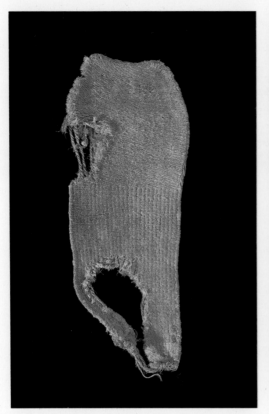
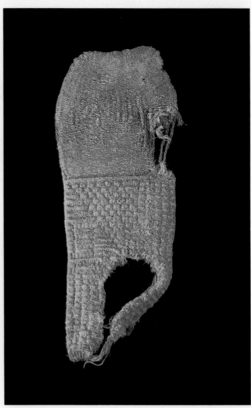

Catalog no.: 692

Site: Sega at Sosa (Tsegi Hatsosie) Canyon, Arizona

Collector and date: Byron Cummings, University of
    Utah Expedition, 1909

Cultural period: Basketmaker III

Construction technique: Composite

Dimensions: Length 20.53 cm, width 10.11 cm,
    depth 0.69 cm

Active elements: Cordage, 2 ply, z-S twist

Average width: 0.11 cm

Passive elements: Cordage, 2 ply, z-S twist

Number of passive units: 28

Number in unit: 1 (except where doubled at toe)

Average width: 0.17 cm

Ties, loops, attachments: Toe: Holes and worn wefts
    show evidence of loops. Heel: Cordage, plug
    remnants. Cord across heel 3 ply, z-S twist

Shape: Right(?) foot shaping. Scalloped toe, heel
    disarticulating

Start: Scalloped toe start

Body: 2/2 alternate pair twining over doubled warps
    for forward one-third section of sandal at which
    point doubled warps end. Remaining length of
    sandal to heel woven in raised geometric pattern

Finish: Heel finish incomplete, but at remnant edge
    warps wrap around group of 2 or 3 cords,
    holding ends down with next wrap. Ends are cut
    off close.

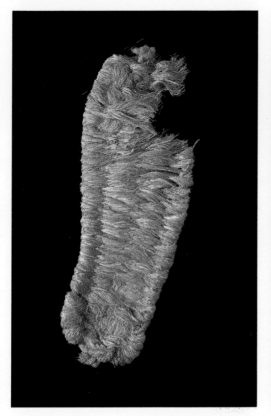
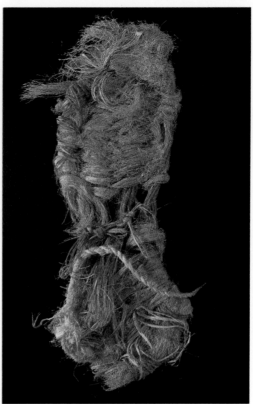

Catalog no.: 732
Site: Sega at Sosa (Tsegi Hatsosie) Canyon, Arizona
Collector and date: Byron Cummings, University of
    Utah Expedition, 1909
Cultural period: Unknown
Construction technique: Plain weave
Dimensions: Length 24.0 cm, width 9.5 cm, depth
    1.4 cm
Active elements: Shredded leaf element unspun,
    partially decorticated
Average width: 0.50 cm
Passive elements: Cordage, 2 ply, s-Z twist
Number of passive units: 4
Number in unit: 1
Average width: 0.60 cm
Ties, loops, attachments: None apparent
Shape: Right foot shaping, rounded heel
Start: Unknown, disarticulating
Body: Over-under plain weave for length of sandal
Finish: At heel warp ends are knotted in two knots
    and tucked back into sandal.
Other: Reinforcement stitches on toe area and heel

Catalog no.: 733.2
Site: Sega at Sosa (Tsegi Hatsosie) Canyon, Arizona
Collector and date: Byron Cummings, University of
    Utah Expedition, 1909
Cultural period: Unknown
Construction technique: Plain weave
Dimensions: Length 32.50 cm, width 10.57 cm,
    depth 1.55 cm
Active elements: Shredded leaf element unspun,
    decorticated
Average width: 0.48 cm
Passive elements: Cordage, 2 ply, z-S twist
Number of passive units: 4
Number in unit: 1
Average width: 0.74 cm
Ties, loops, attachments: Toe: Leaf element loops
    over toe, stitches into sandal, and emerges again
    to double back over toe and stitch into sandal
    and is tied in a double knot.Heel: Fine yucca
    cordage 2 ply s-Z twist tied to each side of
    sandal. One knot is exposed while the other is
    covered by weft. Ends of cordage appear dipped
    in resin.
Shape: Rounded toe and squared heel
Start: Unknown, sandal disarticulating
Body: Over-under plain weave
Finish: Unknown
Other: Mends at heel appear to be holding it
    together.

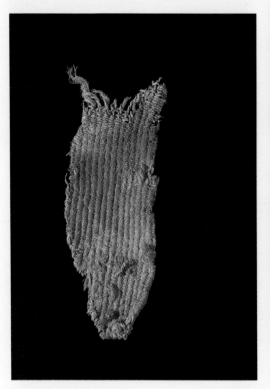

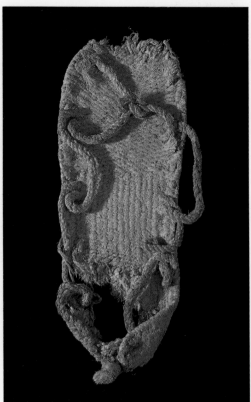

Catalog no.: 741
Site: Sega at Sosa (Tsegi Hatsosie) Canyon, Arizona
Collector and date: Byron Cummings, University of
  Utah Expedition, 1909
Cultural period: Basketmaker III (?)
Construction technique: Plain weave and twined
Dimensions: Length 25.0 cm, width 10.5 cm, depth
  0.8 cm
Active elements: Cordage, 2 ply, z-S twist
Average width: 0.324 cm
Passive elements: Cordage, 2 ply, z-S twist
Number of passive units: 20
Number in unit: 1 (except where doubled at toe)
Average width: 0.45 cm
Ties, loops, attachments: All cordage 3 ply Z twist
  (each ply 2 ply, z-S twist). Toe: Cordage, on left
  side. Edge: Side cords looped through body of
  sandal. Heel: Warp cordage crosses and stitches
  into heel.
Shape: Scalloped toe and puckered heel
Start: Scalloped toe start
Body: 2/2 alternate pair twining over doubled warps
  at toe area. Instep to heel 1/1 plain weave.
Finish: Puckered heel. Overhand knot with warps at
  heel
Other: Perimeter is reinforced with a cordage
  running stitch.

124   *Catalog no.:* 740
    Site: Sega at Sosa (Tsegi Hatsosie) Canyon, Arizona
    Collector and date: Byron Cummings, University of
      Utah Expedition, 1909
    Cultural period: Unknown
    Construction technique: Plain weave
    Dimensions: Length 21.0 cm, width 8.0 cm, depth
      0.53 cm
    Active elements: Cordage, 2 ply, z-S twist
    Average width: 0.12 cm
    Passive elements: Cordage, 2 ply, z-S twist
    Number of passive units: 16
    Number in unit: 1
    Average width: 0.22 cm
    Ties, loops, attachments: Heel: Fragmentary cordage
      2 ply z-S twist. Edge: Fragmentary cordage 2 ply
      z-S twist
    Shape: Unknown, fragmentary
    Start: Missing
    Body: Over-under plain weave for length of
      fragment
    Finish: Missing

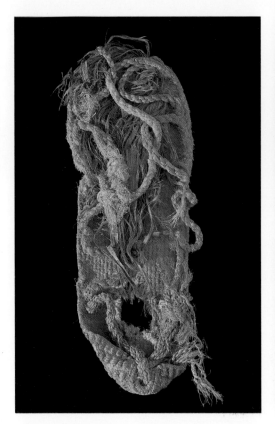

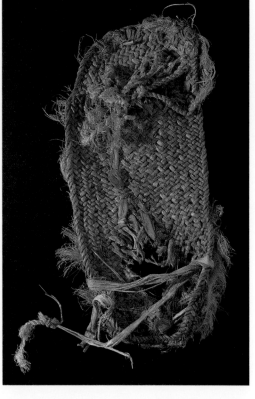

Catalog no.: 744
Site: Sega at Sosa (Tsegi Hatsosie) Canyon, Arizona
Collector and date: Byron Cummings, University of
Utah Expedition, 1909
Cultural period: Basketmaker III
Construction technique: Composite
Dimensions: Length 29.0 cm, width 11.2 cm, depth
0.7 cm
Active elements: Cordage, 2 ply, z-S twist
Average width: 0.12 cm
Passive elements: Cordage, 2 ply, z-S twist
Number of passive units: 28
Number in unit: 1 (except where doubled at toe)
Average width: 0.30 cm
Ties, loops, attachments: Toe: Cordage, 2 ply, s-Z
twist loop and stitch into body of sandal along
edges. Lacing across toe area over padding. Heel:
5-ply cordage, Z twist (each ply 2 ply, z-S twist).
Shape: Right(?) foot shaping, scalloped toe and
puckered heel
Start: Scalloped toe start
Body: 2/2 alternate pair twining over doubled warps
for forward one-third section of sandal at which
point doubled warps end. Remaining length of
sandal to heel woven in raised geometric pattern
Finish: Puckered heel finish. A group of heel cords
from each edge loop and stitch into sides of the
sandal.
Other: Shredded yucca added on upper surface in
toe area

Catalog no.: 745
Site: Sega at Sosa (Tsegi Hatsosie) Canyon, Arizona
Collector and date: Byron Cummings, University of
Utah Expedition, 1909
Cultural period: Unknown
Construction technique: Plaited
Dimensions: Length 25.0 cm, width 10.5 cm, depth
0.5 cm
Active elements: Leaf element unspun, cortex intact
Average width: 0.31 cm
Passive elements: N/A
Ties, loops, attachments: Toe: Cordage ties 2 ply, s-Z
twist. Heel: Leaf elements stitched across heel
Shape: Left foot shaping, rounded toe and cupped
heel
Start: Toe area missing, assume folded start
Body: 2/2 twill plaiting with 2/3/2 at selvage. Shaping
at toe with shifts 2/1/2/2 and 2/2/3/2/2. Ends
frayed on sole for padding
Finish: At heel elements are pulled tight to create
cupped heel.
Other: Sandal appears mended down center and
over toe with leaf element.

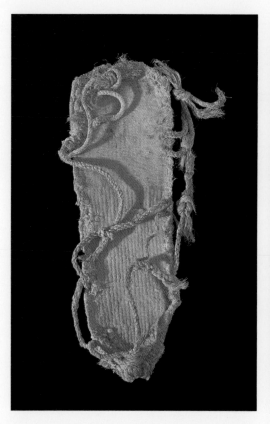
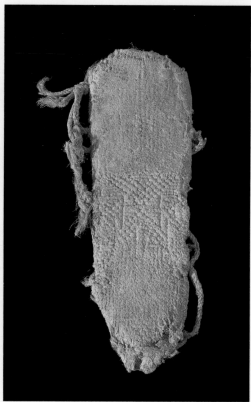

Catalog no.: 746
Site: Sega at Sosa (Tsegi Hatsosie) Canyon, Arizona
Collector and date: Byron Cummings, University of
    Utah Expedition, 1909
Cultural period: Basketmaker III
Construction technique: Composite
Dimensions: Length 26.0 cm, width 9.0 cm, depth
    0.58 cm
Active elements: Cordage, 2 ply, z-S twist
Average width: 0.09 cm
Passive elements: Cordage, 3 ply, z-S twist
Number of passive units: 26
Number in unit: 1 (except where doubled at toe)
Average width: 0.13 cm
Ties, loops, attachments: Toe: Plug remnants. Heel:
    Two heel cords 3 ply, Z twist (each ply 2 ply z-S
    twist) loop and stitch into sandal on both sides
    and connect to edge cords. Edge: Loop cordage
    3 ply, Z twist (each ply 2 ply z-S twist) loop and
    stitch into body of sandal along both edges.
    Cordage, added with knots.
Shape: Left(?) foot shaping, scalloped toe and
    puckered heel
Start: Scalloped toe start
Body: 2/2 alternate pair twining over doubled warps
    for forward one-third section of sandal at which
    point doubled warps end. Remaining length of
    sandal woven in raised geometric pattern
Finish: Puckered heel finish. Heel cords gathered
    together and wrapped before separating into
    two cords

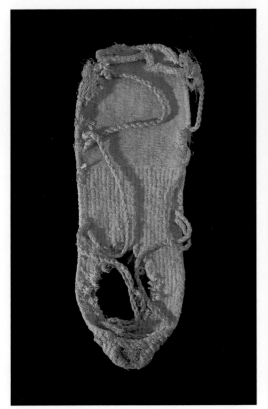
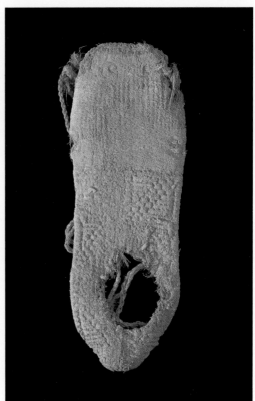

Catalog no.: 747
Site: Sega at Sosa (Tsegi Hatsosie) Canyon, Arizona
Collector and date: Byron Cummings, University of
    Utah Expedition, 1909
Cultural period: Basketmaker III
Construction technique: Composite
Dimensions: Length 26.5 cm, width 11.5 cm, depth
    0.5 cm
Active elements: Cordage, 2 ply, z-S twist
Average width: 0.14 cm
Passive elements: Cordage, 3 ply, z-S twist
Number of passive units: 26
Number in unit: 1 (except where doubled at toe)
Average width: 0.25 cm
Ties, loops, attachments: Toe: Cordage, 2 ply, Z twist
    (each ply 2 ply z-S twist). Edges: Ties looped and
    stitched into body of sandal. Right edge 2 ply,
    s-Z twist. Left edge 2 ply, Z twist (each ply 2 ply,
    z-S twist). Heel: Cordage, 2 ply, Z twist (each ply
    2 ply z-S twist), connects to edge loops
Shape: Rounded toe (probably scalloped before
    wear) and puckered heel
Start: Scalloped toe start
Body: 2/2 alternate pair twining over doubled warps
    for forward one-third of sandal, at which point
    doubled warps end. Remaining length of sandal
    to heel woven in raised geometric pattern
Finish: Puckered heel finish. Heel cords cross and
    stitch into body of sandal and continue as edge
    cords.

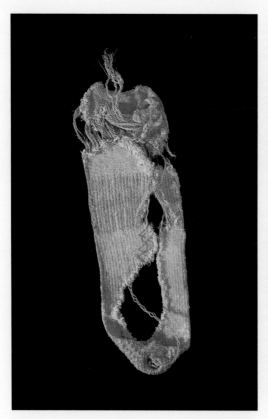
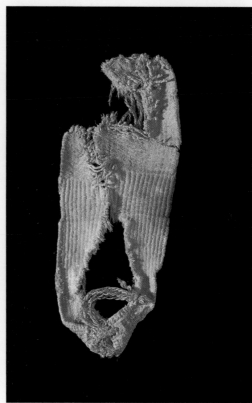

128
Catalog no.: 754
Site: Sega at Sosa (Tsegi Hatsosie) Canyon, Arizona
Collector and date: Byron Cummings, University of
Utah Expedition, 1909
Cultural period: Basketmaker III
Construction technique: Composite
Dimensions: Length 24.8 cm, width 8.0 cm, depth
0.45 cm
Active elements: Cordage, 2 ply, z-S twist
Average width: 0.09 cm
Passive elements: Cordage, 3 ply, z-S twist
Number of passive units: 30
Number in unit: 1 (except where doubled at toe)
Average width: 0.24 cm
Ties, loops, attachments: Toe: Two remnants of toe
loop, 2 ply, s-Z twist. Heel: Long heel cord 3 ply,
z-S twist.
Shape: Right(?) foot shaping, scalloped toe and
puckered heel
Start: Scalloped toe start
Body: 2/2 alternate pair twining over doubled warps
for forward one-third section of sandal at which
point doubled warps end. Midsection has two
colored bands. One is yellow/orange and the
other is brown(?). Possible geometric design
using A & B weaving. Remaining heel section is
woven in raised geometric pattern.
Finish: Puckered heel finish. Ends tucked to surface
of sandal. Breakage on right side. One long cord
remains.

Catalog no.: 755
Site: Sega at Sosa (Tsegi Hatsosie) Canyon, Arizona
Collector and date: Byron Cummings, University of
Utah Expedition, 1909
Cultural period: Basketmaker III
Construction technique: Composite
Dimensions: Length 23.5 cm, width 9.5 cm, depth
0.67 cm
Active elements: Cordage, 2 ply, z-S twist
Average width: 0.08 cm
Passive elements: Cordage, element 3 ply, z-S twist
Number of passive units: 26
Number in unit: 1 (except where doubled at toe)
Average width: 0.30 cm
Ties, loops, attachments: Heel: Five-six cords are 3
ply, z-S twist. Wrapped at end
Shape: Scalloped toe and puckered heel
Start: Scalloped toe start
Body: 2/2 alternate pair twining over doubled warps
for forward one-third section of sandal at which
point doubled warps end. Midsection appears to
have a dyed weft pattern. Remaining length of
sandal to heel woven in raised geometric pattern
Finish: Puckered heel finish. Heel cords are
gathered together and wrapped with a 3 ply, s-Z
twist cord on upper surface of sandal.

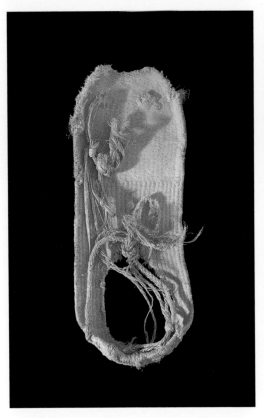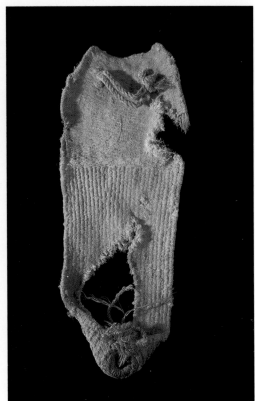

Catalog no.: 756
Site: Sega at Sosa (Tsegi Hatsosie) Canyon, Arizona
Collector and date: Byron Cummings, University of
Utah Expedition, 1909
Cultural period: Basketmaker III
Construction technique: Composite
Dimensions: Length 24.0 cm, width 9.7 cm, depth
0.35 cm
Active elements: Cordage, 2 ply, z-S twist
Average width: 0.15 sm
Passive elements: Cordage, 3 ply, z-S twist
Number of passive units: 26
Number in unit: 1 (except where doubled at toe)
Average width: 0.15 cm
Ties, loops, attachments: Toe: Knot remnants. Leaf
element from left side of toe extends and loops
around ankle. Heel: Four cords, 3 ply, z-S twist,
plus remnants of possible ties. Three cords
knotted to ankle loop are 3 ply, Z twist (each
ply 2 ply z-S twist).
Shape: Left(?) foot shaping, scalloped toe and
puckered heel
Start: Scalloped toe start
Body: 2/2 alternate pair twining over doubled warps
for forward one-third section of sandal at which
point doubled warps end. Remaining length of
sandal to heel woven in raised geometric pattern
Finish: Puckered heel finish. Warp ends neatly
stitched at heel in herringbone
Other: Mend at toe using leaf element

Catalog no.: 757
Site: Sega at Sosa (Tsegi Hatsosie) Canyon, Arizona
Collector and date: Byron Cummings, University of
Utah Expedition, 1909
Cultural period: Basketmaker III
Construction technique: Composite
Dimensions: Length 26.0 cm, width 10.5 cm, depth
0.65 cm
Active elements: Cordage, 2 ply, z-S twist
Average width: 0.13 cm
Passive elements: Cordage, 3 ply, z-S twist
Number of passive units: 30
Number in unit: 1 (except where doubled at toe)
Average width: 0.17 cm
Ties, loops, attachments: Toe: Two cords 3 ply, Z
twist (each ply 2 ply, z-S twist) form toe loop.
One loop knotted. Heel: Two cord fragments 3
ply, Z twist (each ply 2 ply, z-S twist)
Shape: Left(?) foot shaping, scalloped toe and
puckered heel
Start: Scalloped toe start
Body: 2/2 alternate pair twining over doubled warps
for forward one-third section of sandal at which
point doubled warps end. Remaining length of
sandal woven in raised geometric pattern
Finish: Puckered heel finish. Heel cords missing
except for two ties extending from each side

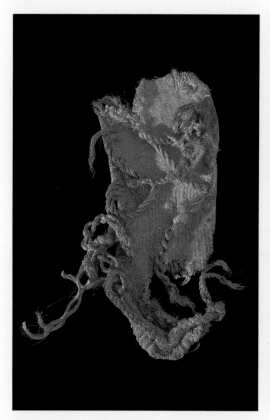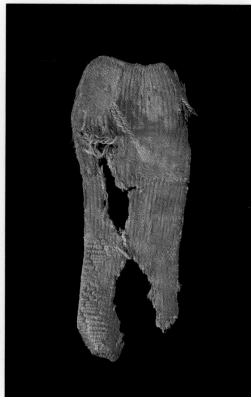

130 *Catalog no.:* 760

Site: Sega at Sosa (Tsegi Hatsosie) Canyon, Arizona

Collector and date: Byron Cummings, University of Utah Expedition, 1909

Cultural period: Basketmaker III

Construction technique: Composite

Dimensions: Length 26.5 cm, width 12.0 cm, depth 0.60 cm

Active elements: Cordage, 2 ply, z-S twist

Average width: 0.13 cm

Passive elements: Cordage, 2 ply, z-S twist

Number of passive units: 28 or 29

Number in unit: 1 (except where doubled at toe)

Average width: 0.70 cm

Ties, loops, attachments: Heel: Cordage, 3 ply, Z twist (each ply 2 ply, z-S twist). Edges: Five different types of cordage laced at edges: 3 ply, s-Z twist; 2 ply, z-S twist; 2 ply, S twist (each ply 2 ply, s-Z twist); 2 ply, Z twist (each ply 2 ply z-S twist); 2 ply, s-Z twist.

Shape: Right(?) foot shaping, scalloped toe and puckered heel

Start: Scalloped toe start

Body: 2/2 alternate pair twining over doubled warps for forward one-third section of sandal at which point doubled warps end. Remaining length of sandal to heel woven in raised geometric pattern

Finish: Puckered heel finish. Two groups of warp heel cords tucked to inside then extend on both sides of sandal to connect with edge ties.

Other: Running stitch along both edges from toe to just past instep

Catalog no.: 761

Site: Sega at Sosa (Tsegi Hatsosie) Canyon, Arizona

Collector and date: Byron Cummings, University of Utah Expedition, 1909

Cultural period: Basketmaker III

Construction technique: Composite

Dimensions: Length 25.0 cm, width 10.0 cm, depth 1.10 cm

Active elements: Cordage, 2 ply, z-S twist

Average width: 0.11 cm

Passive elements: Cordage, 3 ply, z-S twist

Number of passive units: 28(?)

Number in unit: 1 (except where doubled at toe)

Average width: 0.14 cm

Ties, loops, attachments: Toe: Remnants of ties, one loop attachment

Shape: Right(?) foot shaping, scalloped toe, heel missing

Start: Scalloped toe start

Body: 2/2 alternate pair twining over doubled warps for forward one-third section of sandal at which point doubled warps end. Midsection is woven on single elements in a probable geometric design but is too worn to determine. Remaining length of sandal to heel woven in raised geometric pattern

Finish: Missing

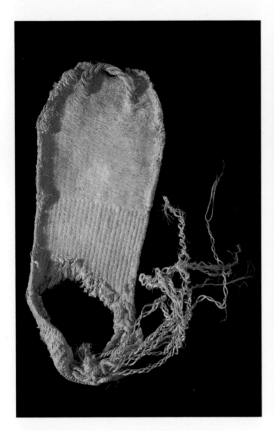

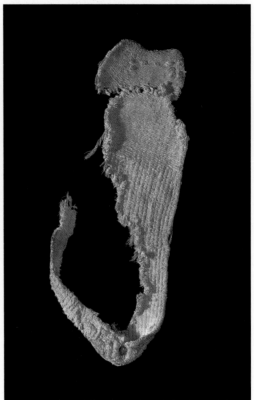

Catalog no.: 762
Site: Sega at Sosa (Tsegi Hatsosie) Canyon, Arizona
Collector and date: Byron Cummings, University of
 Utah Expedition, 1909
Cultural period: Basketmaker III
Construction technique: Composite
Dimensions: Length 25.54 cm, width 10.02 cm,
 depth 0.50 cm
Active elements: Cordage, 2 ply, z-S twist
Average width: 0.12 cm
Passive elements: Cordage, 3 ply, z-S twist
Number of passive units: 24
Number in unit: 1 (except where doubled at toe)
Average width: 0.13 cm
Ties, loops, attachments: Toe: Loop cordage 3 ply, z-S
 twist. Heel: Cordage, 3 ply, z-S twist
Shape: Scalloped toe and puckered heel
Start: Scalloped toe start
Body: 2/2 alternate pair twining over doubled warps
 for forward one-third section of sandal at which
 point doubled warps end. Remaining length of
 sandal woven in raised geometric pattern
Finish: Puckered heel finish. After gathering in heel
 cords they cross and knot. One half of cords
 appear cut while the other half extend
 untwisted.
Other: Mend on right side of heel with cordage 2
 ply, s-Z twist. One tie forms mend loops around
 heel cord.

Catalog no.: 763
Site: Sega at Sosa (Tsegi Hatsosie) Canyon, Arizona
Collector and date: Byron Cummings, University of
 Utah Expedition, 1909
Cultural period: Basketmaker III
Construction technique: Composite
Dimensions: Length 25.5 cm, width 8.1 cm, depth
 0.66 cm
Active elements: Cordage, 2 ply, z-S twist
Average width: 0.13 sm
Passive elements: Cordage, 3 ply, z-S twist
Number of passive units: 20
Number in unit: 1 (except where doubled at toe)
Average width: 0.18 cm
Ties, loops, attachments: Toe: Loop remnants
Shape: Scalloped toe and puckered heel
Start: Scalloped toe start
Body: 2/2 alternate pair twining over doubled warps
 for forward one-third section of sandal at which
 point doubled warps end. Remaining length of
 sandal to heel woven in raised geometric pattern
Finish: Puckered heel finish. Ends missing

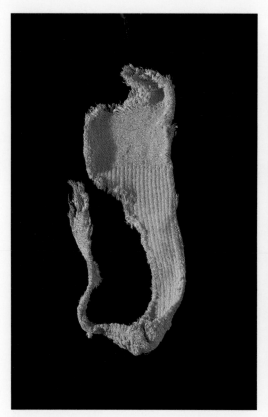
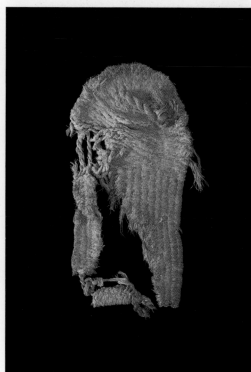

132

Catalog no.: 764
Site: Sega at Sosa (Tsegi Hatsosie) Canyon, Arizona
Collector and date: Byron Cummings, University of
Utah Expedition, 1909
Cultural period: Basketmaker III
Construction technique: Composite
Dimensions: Length 23.5 cm, width 8.5 cm, depth
0.69 cm
Active elements: Cordage, 2 ply, z-S twist
Average width: 0.12 cm
Passive elements: Cordage, 3 ply, z-S twist
Number of passive units: 22
Number in unit: 1 (except where doubled at toe)
Average width: 0.18 cm
Ties, loops, attachments: Edge: Remnant on right
edge (or stitching)
Shape: Possible scalloped toe and puckered heel
Start: Scalloped toe start
Body: 2/2 alternate pair twining over doubled warps
for forward one-third section of sandal at which
point doubled warps end. Midsection woven on
single warps. Pattern is too worn to determine.
Remainder of sandal woven in raised geometric
pattern
Finish: Puckered heel finish

Catalog no.: 765
Site: Sega at Sosa (Tsegi Hatsosie) Canyon, Arizona
Collector and date: Byron Cummings, University of
Utah Expedition, 1909
Cultural period: Basketmaker III
Construction technique: Plain weave and twined
Dimensions: Length 22.0 cm, width 11.5 cm, depth
0.63 cm
Active elements: Cordage, 2 ply, z-S twist
Average width: 0.24 cm
Passive elements: Cordage, 2 ply, z-S twist
Number of passive units: 14
Number in unit: 1
Average width: 0.31 cm
Ties, loops, attachments: Toe: Loop of cordage 2 ply,
s-Z twist knotted through sandal. Heel: Fragment
of leaf element knot
Shape: Left(?) foot shaping, rounded toe, heel
missing
Start: Seven cordage warps folded at toe (one
inside the other) to form 14 warps. Weft
cordage woven tightly at start to round toe
Body: 2/2 alternate pair twining for forward one-
third section of sandal. Remainder of sandal is
woven 1/1 plain weave.
Finish: Missing

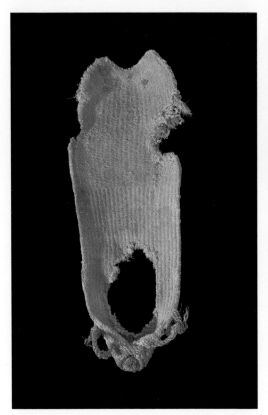 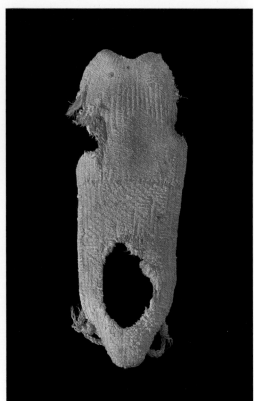

Catalog no.: 908
Site: Sega at Sosa (Tsegi Hatsosie) Canyon, Arizona
Collector and date: Byron Cummings, University of
    Utah Expedition, 1909
Cultural period: Basketmaker III
Construction technique: Composite
Dimensions: Length 26.2 cm, width 10.0 cm, depth
    0.80 cm
Active elements: Cordage, 2 ply, z-S twist
Average width: 0.13 cm
Passive elements: Cordage, 3 ply, z-S twist
Number of passive units: 26
Number in unit: 1 (except where doubled at toe)
Average width: 0.25 cm
Ties, loops, attachments: Toe: Remnants of ties. Heel:
    Warp cordage on both sides, 3 ply, Z twist (each
    ply 3 ply, z-S twist).
Shape: Scalloped toe and puckered heel
Start: Scalloped toe start
Body: 2/2 alternate pair twining over doubled warps
    for forward one-third section of sandal at which
    point doubled warps end. Remaining two-thirds
    of sandal woven in raised geometric pattern
Finish: Puckered heel finish. Warp heel cords
    extend from both sides of heel, loop, and knot
    into sandal.

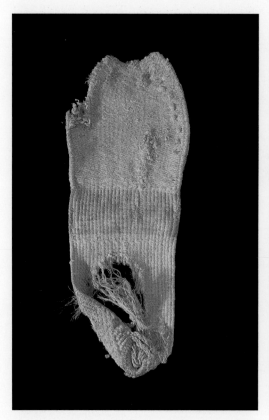
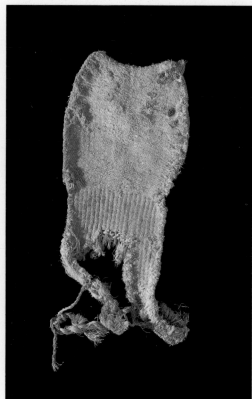

134 Catalog no.: 909

Site: Sega at Sosa (Tsegi Hatsosie) Canyon, Arizona
Collector and date: Byron Cummings, University of
  Utah Expedition, 1909
Cultural period: Basketmaker III
Construction technique: Composite
Dimensions: Length 26.45 cm, width 10.53 cm,
  depth 0.80 cm
Active elements: Cordage, 2 ply, z-S twist
Average width: 0.12 cm
Passive elements: Cordage, 3 ply, z-S twist
Number of passive units: 30
Number in unit: 1 (except where doubled at toe)
Average width: 0.19 cm
Ties, loops, attachments: Toe: Loop remnants. Heel:
  Warp ties, 3 ply Z twist cordage (each ply 2 ply,
  z-S twist)
Shape: Scalloped toe and puckered heel
Start: Scalloped toe start
Body: 2/2 alternate pair twining over doubled warps
  for forward one-third section of sandal at which
  point doubled warps end. Midsection has one
  band in a red-yellow and natural and a second
  band in a black-gray and natural. Possible
  geometric design in A & B weaving. Remaining
  heel section woven in raised geometric pattern.
Finish: Puckered heel finish. Warp ends tucked
  through heel hole to upper surface where they
  are wrapped and left protruding
Other: Running stitches of cordage on forward right
  edge of sandal

Catalog no.: 910
Site: Sega at Sosa (Tsegi Hatsosie) Canyon, Arizona
Collector and date: Byron Cummings, University of
  Utah Expedition, 1909
Cultural period: Basketmaker III
Construction technique: Composite
Dimensions: Length 20.2 cm, width 9.89 cm, depth
  1.00 cm
Active elements: Cordage, 2 ply, z-S twist
Average width: 0.09 cm
Passive elements: Cordage, 3 ply, z-S twist
Number of passive units: 22
Number in unit: 1 (except where doubled at toe)
Average width: 0.23 cm
Ties, loops, attachments: Edge: Remnants of side
  loops. Heel: Heavy cord 2 ply s-Z twist knotted.
  Fine cordage 2 ply s-Z twist. Knot on right side
  of sole
Shape: Scalloped toe, heel missing
Start: Scalloped toe start
Body: 2/2 alternate pair twining over doubled warps
  for forward one-third section of sandal at which
  point doubled warps end. Remaining length of
  sandal to heel woven in raised geometric pattern
Finish: Missing
Other: Running stitches appear on both sides of toe
  area.

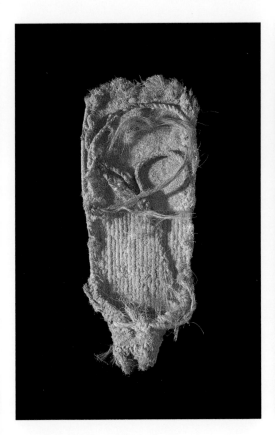

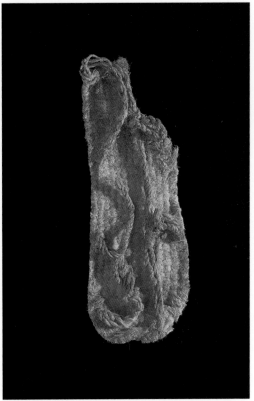

Catalog no.: 911
Site: Sega at Sosa (Tsegi Hatsosie) Canyon, Arizona
Collector and date: Byron Cummings, University of
   Utah Expedition, 1909
Cultural period: Basketmaker III
Construction technique: Composite
Dimensions: Length 23.8 cm, width 9.9 cm, depth
   1.20 cm
Active elements: Cordage, 2 ply, z-S twist
Average width: 0.15 cm
Passive elements: Cordage, 3 ply, z-S twist
Number of passive units: 26
Number in unit: 1 (except where doubled at toe)
Average width: 0.19 cm
Ties, loops, attachments: Toe: Remnants. Heel:
   Cordage, 2 ply, s-Z twist. Edge: Ties of cordage,
   2 ply Z twist (each ply 2 ply s-Z twist). One tie
   of 3 ply, s-Z twist on left side
Shape: Left(?) foot shaping, scalloped toe and
   puckered heel
Start: Scalloped toe start
Body: 2/2 alternate pair twining over doubled warps
   for forward one-third section of sandal at which
   point doubled warps end. Remaining length of
   sandal to heel woven in raised geometric pattern
Finish: Puckered heel finish. End missing. Heel
   knotted
Other: Mending at heel

Catalog no.: 916
Site: Sega at Sosa (Tsegi Hatsosie) Canyon, Arizona
Collector and date: Byron Cummings, University of
   Utah Expedition, 1909
Cultural period: Basketmaker III (?)
Construction technique: Plain weave and twined
Dimensions: Length 22.0 cm, width 8.4 cm, depth
   0.72 cm
Active elements: Cordage, 2 ply, z-S twist
Average width: 0.24 cm
Passive elements: Cordage, 2 ply, z-S twist
Number of passive units: 14
Number in unit: 1
Average width: 0.55 cm
Ties, loops, attachments: Toe: Toe loop remnant.
   Heel: Two-ply heel cords twisted Z (each ply 2
   ply, z-S twist). Edge: Cords extend from toe,
   loop, and stitch into sides of sandal and attach to
   heel cords. Cords are 2 ply, Z twist (each ply 2
   ply, z-s twist).
Shape: Left foot shaping, heart shaped toe, heel is
   fragmentary but appears puckered.
Start: Seven warps appear folded at toe (one inside
   the other or possibly crossing) to form 14
   warps. Twining or plain weave at start woven
   very tight
Body: It appears there are 3-4 rows of plain weave
   followed by a row of three-element twining for
   length of sandal.
Finish: Puckered heel finish. Heel cords attach to
   edge cords.

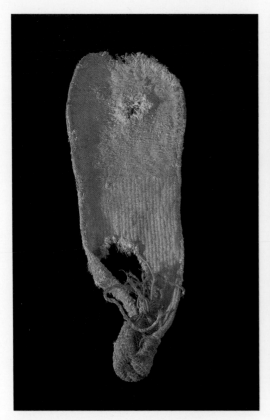 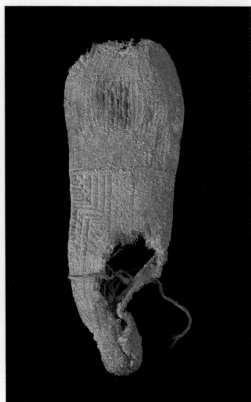

Catalog no.: 912
Site: Sega at Sosa (Tsegi Hatsosie) Canyon, Arizona
Collector and date: Byron Cummings, University of
    Utah Expedition, 1909
Cultural period: Basketmaker III
Construction technique: Composite
Dimensions: Length 27.5 cm, width 10.2 cm, depth
    0.87 cm
Active elements: Cordage, 2 ply, z-S twist
Average width: 0.09 cm
Passive elements: Cordage, 3 ply, z-S twist
Number of passive units: 30(?)
Number in unit: 1 (except where doubled at toe)
Average width: 0.14 cm
Ties, loops, attachments: Toe: Cordage, remnants.
    Heel: Unattached cordage, 2 ply (s-Z twist)
    loops around damaged heel section. Possible heel
    cord emerges on left side, knotted with 5-6 fine
    cords, 2 ply z-S twist.
Shape: Scalloped toe and puckered heel
Start: Scalloped toe start
Body: 2/2 alternate pair twining over doubled warps
    for forward one-third section of sandal at which
    point doubled warps end. Remaining length of
    sandal to heel woven in raised geometric pattern
Finish: Puckered heel finish. Ends appear tucked to
    inside.
Other: Running stitches on both sides of forward
    one-third section of sandal

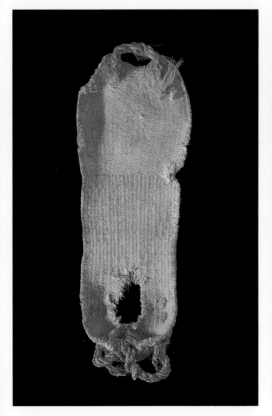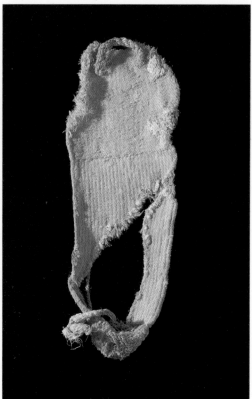

Catalog no.: 978
Site: Sega at Sosa (Tsegi Hatsosie) Canyon, Arizona
Collector and date: Byron Cummings, University of
  Utah Expedition, 1909
Cultural period: Basketmaker III
Construction technique: Composite
Dimensions: Length 22.5 cm, width 10.0 cm, depth
  0.60 cm
Active elements: Cordage, 2 ply, z-S twist
Average width: 0.09 cm
Passive elements: Cordage, 3 ply, z-S twist
Number of passive units: 26
Number in unit: 1 (except where doubled at toe)
Average width: 0.27 cm
Ties, loops, attachments: Toe: Cordage, 2 ply Z twist
  (each ply 2 ply, z-S twist). Heel: Fine cordage 2
  ply, s-Z twist and heavier cordage 3 ply, s-Z
  twist. Edge: Possible loop fragments
Shape: Scalloped toe and puckered heel
Start: Scalloped toe start
Body: 2/2 alternate pair twining over doubled warps
  for forward one-third section of sandal at which
  point doubled warps end. Remaining two-thirds
  of sandal woven in raised geometric pattern
Finish: Puckered heel finish. Heel cords cross each
  other and loop back, stitching into sandal.

Catalog no.: 979
Site: Sega at Sosa (Tsegi Hatsosie) Canyon, Arizona
Collector and date: Byron Cummings, University of
  Utah Expedition, 1909
Cultural period: Basketmaker III
Construction technique: Composite
Dimensions: Length 25.0 cm, width 9.5 cm, depth
  0.55 cm
Active elements: Cordage, 2 ply, z-S twist
Average width: 0.10 cm
Passive elements: Cordage, 3 ply, z-S twist
Number of passive units: 30
Number in unit: 1 (except where doubled at toe)
Average width: 0.17 cm
Ties, loops, attachments: Toe: Cordage, loop 2 ply z
  twist. One ply single, the other ply 2 ply (each
  ply 3 ply z-S twist). Heel: Cordage, fragment 3
  ply, z twist (each ply 3 ply z-S twist). Edge:
  Knotted and looped cordage 2 ply, s-Z twist
  (each ply z-S twist).
Shape: Right(?) foot shaping, scalloped toe and
  puckered heel
Start: Scalloped toe start
Body: 2/2 alternate pair twining over doubled warps
  for forward one-third section of sandal at which
  point doubled warps end. Remaining two-thirds
  of sandal woven in raised geometric pattern
Finish: Puckered heel finish. Warp ends pushed
  through heel hole to back of sandal

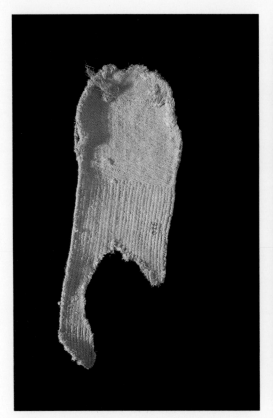
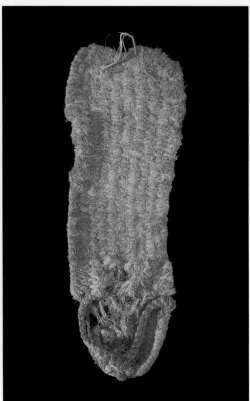

138   Catalog no.: 980
       Site: Sega at Sosa (Tsegi Hatsosie) Canyon, Arizona
       Collector and date: Byron Cummings, University of
           Utah Expedition, 1909
       Cultural period: Basketmaker III
       Construction technique: Composite
       Dimensions: Length 24.5 cm, width 9.0 cm, depth
           0.54 cm
       Active elements: Cordage, 2 ply, z-S twist
       Average width: 0.10 cm
       Passive elements: Cordage, 3 ply, z-S twist
       Number of passive units: 30
       Number in unit: 1 (except where doubled at toe)
       Average width: 0.15 cm
       Ties, loops, attachments: Toe: Cordage, 2 or 3 ply,
           z-S twist, remnants at four points in toe area
       Shape: Right(?) foot shaping, scalloped toe and heel
           missing
       Start: Scalloped toe start
       Body: 2/2 alternate pair twining over doubled warps
           for forward one-third section of sandal at which
           point doubled warps end. Remaining length of
           sandal to heel woven in raised geometric pattern
       Finish: Heel missing

Catalog no.: 982
Site: Sega at Sosa (Tsegi Hatsosie) Canyon, Arizona
Collector and date: Byron Cummings, University of
    Utah Expedition, 1909
Cultural period: Unknown
Construction technique: Plain weave
Dimensions: Length 27.5 cm, width 10.0 cm, depth
    1.10 cm
Active elements: Cordage, 2 ply, z-S twist
Average width: 0.43 cm
Passive elements: Cordage, 2 ply, z-S twist
Number of passive units: 10(?)
Number in unit: 1
Average width: 0.49 cm
Ties, loops, attachments: Toe: Broken leaf element.
    Heel: Heel loop cordage 2 ply, Z twist (each ply
    2 ply z-S twist) is attached on one edge only.
Shape: Left foot shaping, heart-shaped toe and
    puckered heel
Start: It appears 5(?) warps were folded at toe to
    form 10(?) warps. The arrangement appears to
    be that edge warps cross over each other at the
    center; another warp folds at center crossing the
    first two warps; and two warps are folded (one
    on each side) inside the outer edge warp.
Body: Over-under plain weave from toe to heel
Finish: Puckered heel finish. Two warps from each
    side become the heel cord which the remaining
    warps wrap around. Heel cord from right side is
    brought between 2 warps from left side. Both
    heel cords are 2 ply Z twist (each ply 2 ply z-S
    twist).

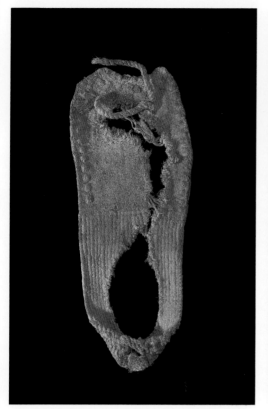 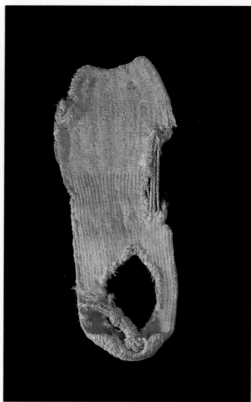

Catalog no.: 983
Site: Sega at Sosa (Tsegi Hatsosie) Canyon, Arizona
Collector and date: Byron Cummings, University of
    Utah Expedition, 1909
Cultural period: Basketmaker III
Construction technique: Composite
Dimensions: Length 25.5 cm, width 10.5 cm, depth
    0.65 cm
Active elements: Cordage, 2 ply, z-S twist
Average width: 0.12 cm
Passive elements: Cordage, 3 ply, z-S twist
Number of passive units: 26
Number in unit: 1 (except where doubled at toe)
Average width: 0.19 cm
Ties, loops, attachments: Toe: Two loops, one intact
    and one detached, of cordage 3 ply, s-Z twist.
    Heel: Cords at heel are bound together with
    wrapping and emerge as a tassel.
Shape: Right foot shaping, scalloped toe and
    puckered heel
Start: Scalloped toe start
Body: 2/2 alternate pair twining over doubled warps
    for almost half of sandal at which point doubled
    warps end. Yellow ochre appears as a wide band
    of color on lower section of 2/2 twining.
    Midsection is woven in a stepped design of two
    bands using different dyed wefts. The first band
    toward the toe is a brown-gray and the second
    band a yellow-gold. Sole is too worn to
    determine weave. Heel section woven in raised
    geometric pattern
Finish: Puckered heel finish. Warp groups from each
    side cross each other, are wrapped, and extend
    through heel hole like a tassel.
Other: Running stitches along forward section of

sandal on both edges. Yellow and red dye on
both surfaces of sandal

Catalog no.: 981
Site: Sega at Sosa (Tsegi Hatsosie) Canyon, Arizona
Collector and date: Byron Cummings, University of
    Utah Expedition, 1909
Cultural period: Basketmaker III
Construction technique: Composite
Dimensions: Length 25.5 cm, width 10.7 cm, depth
    1.8 cm
Active elements: Cordage, 2 ply, z-S twist
Average width: 0.88 cm
Passive elements: Cordage, 3 ply, z-S twist
Number of passive units: 30
Number in unit: 1 (except where doubled at toe)
Average width: 0.17 cm
Ties, loops, attachments: Toe: Two remnants of ties.
    Heel: Two remnants of ties
Shape: Left(?) foot shaping, scalloped toe and
    puckered heel
Start: Scalloped toe start
Body: 2/2 alternate pair twining over doubled warps
    for forward one-third section of sandal at which
    point doubled warps end. Two bands of color at
    midsection. Top band is yellow and bottom band
    is yellow, brown(?) and natural. Geometric
    design possible using A & B weaving. Heel
    section woven in raised geometric pattern
Finish: Puckered heel finish. Warp cords extending
    from both sides are gathered into one bundle
    and tucked under own wrapping. Bundle is then
    wrapped and knotted at end.

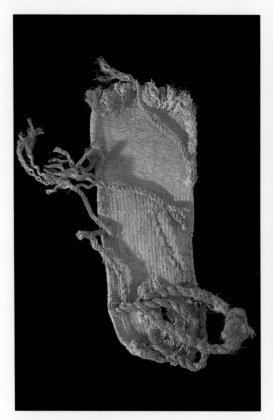
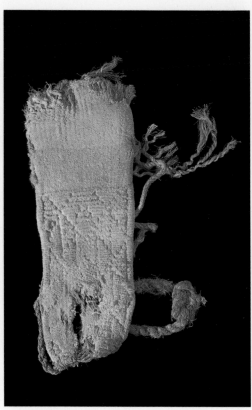

Catalog no.: 985
Site: Sega at Sosa (Tsegi Hatsosie) Canyon, Arizona
Collector and date: Byron Cummings, University of
  Utah Expedition, 1909
Cultural period: Basketmaker III
Construction technique: Composite
Dimensions: Length 23.4 cm, width 9.0 cm, depth
  0.58 cm
Active elements: Cordage, 2 ply, z-S twist
Average width: 0.14 cm
Passive elements: Cordage, 3 ply, z-S twist
Number of passive units: 26
Number in unit: 1 (except where doubled at toe)
Average width: 0.31 cm
Ties, loops, attachments: Toe and Edge: Cordage,
  ties, 3 ply, Z twist (each ply 2 ply, z-S twist) are
  broken at toe, but loop and stitch into sandal
  along edges to heel. Heel: Cordage, loop, 2 ply,
  Z twist (one ply 4 ply z-S twist, and one ply 3
  ply z-S twist). Other: Cordage, loop through
  heel loop is 2 ply Z twist (each ply 2 ply z-s
  twist).
Shape: Left(?) foot shaping, possible scalloped toe
  and puckered heel
Start: Missing, probable scalloped toe start
Body: 2/2 alternate-pair twining over doubled warps
  for forward one-third section of sandal at which
  point doubled warps end. Remaining length of
  sandal to heel woven in raised geometric pattern
Finish: Part of heel missing; probable puckered heel
  finish

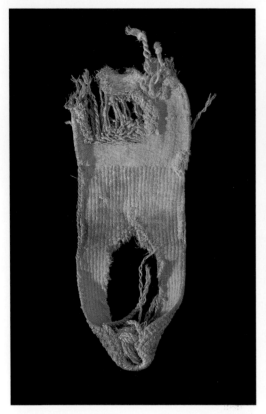

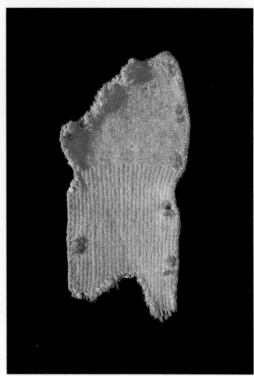

Catalog no.: **986**
Site: Sega at Sosa (Tsegi Hatsosie) Canyon, Arizona
Collector and date: Byron Cummings, University of
Utah Expedition, 1909
Cultural period: Basketmaker III
Construction technique: Composite
Dimensions: Length 25.5 cm, width 10.0 cm, depth
0.4 cm
Active elements: Cordage, 2 ply, z-S twist
Average width: 0.12 cm
Passive elements: Cordage, 3 ply, z-S twist
Number of passive units: 30
Number in unit: 1 (except where doubled at toe)
Average width: 0.25 cm
Ties, loops, attachments: Toe: Cordage, 2 ply, z-S
twist. Heel: Cordage, 3 ply, Z twist (two cords
are each 2 ply, z-S twist, 1 cord is 3 ply z-S
twist)
Shape: Right(?) foot shaping, scalloped toe, and
puckered heel
Start: Scalloped toe start
Body: 2/2 alternate pair twining over doubled warps
for forward one-third section of sandal at which
point doubled warps end. Two bands of color at
midsection. One band is yellow and brown(?);
the other band reddish-brown and yellow.
Remaining length of sandal to heel woven in
raised geometric pattern
Finish: Puckered heel finish. Heel cords cross and
stitch into each side of heel. Remaining warps
tuck to inside of sandal.

Catalog no.: **987**
Site: Sega at Sosa (Tsegi Hatsosie) Canyon, Arizona
Collector and date: Byron Cummings, University of
Utah Expedition, 1909
Cultural period: Basketmaker III
Construction technique: Composite
Dimensions: Length 21.0 cm, width 11.0 cm, depth
0.60 cm
Active elements: Cordage, 2 ply, z-S twist
Average width: 0.02 cm
Passive elements: Cordage, 3 ply, z-S twist
Number of passive units: 26
Number in unit: 1 (except where doubled at toe)
Average width: 0.15 cm
Ties, loops, attachments: Edge: Remnants along both
edges of cordage, 3 ply(?) s-Z twist
Shape: Scalloped toe, heel missing
Start: Scalloped toe start
Body: 2/2 alternate pair twining over doubled warps
for forward one-third section of sandal at which
point doubled warps end. Remaining length of
sandal to heel woven in raised geometric pattern
Finish: Missing

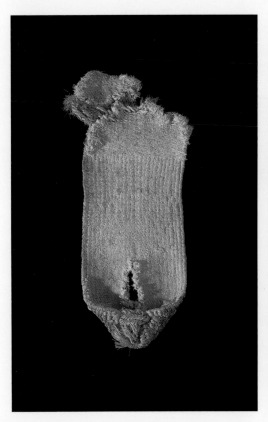
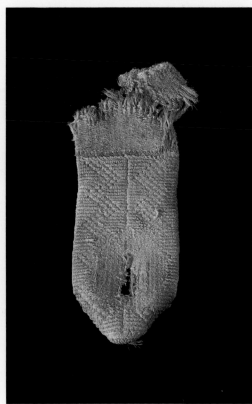

Catalog no.: 989
Site: Sega at Sosa (Tsegi Hatsosie) Canyon, Arizona
Collector and date: Byron Cummings, University of
   Utah Expedition, 1909
Cultural period: Basketmaker III
Construction technique: Composite
Dimensions: Length 23.0 cm, width 11.0 cm, depth
   0.60 cm
Active elements: Cordage, 2 ply, z-S twist
Average width: 0.11 cm
Passive elements: Cordage, 3 ply, z-S twist
Number of passive units: 26
Number in unit: 1 (except where doubled at toe)
Average width: 0.23 cm
Ties, loops, attachments: None apparent
Shape: Scalloped toe, and puckered heel
Start: Scalloped toe start
Body: 2/2 alternate pair twining over doubled warps
   for forward one-third section of sandal at which
   point doubled warps end. Remaining length of
   sandal woven in raised geometric pattern
Finish: Puckered heel finish. Ends tucked to inside

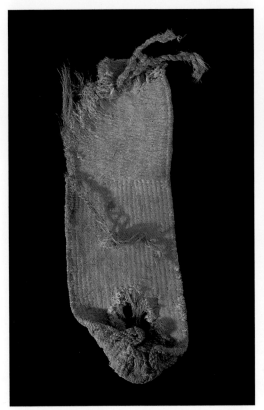
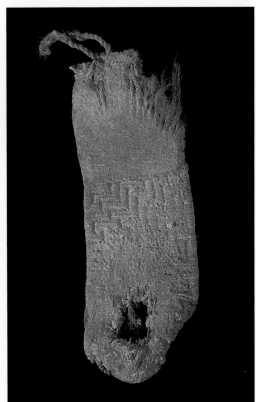

Catalog no.: 3504.1
Site: Sega at Sosa (Tsegi Hatsosie) Canyon, Arizona
Collector and date: Byron Cummings, University of
　Utah Expedition, 1909
Cultural period: Basketmaker III
Construction technique: Composite
Dimensions: Length 27.0 cm, width 9.2 cm, depth
　0.70 cm
Active elements: Cordage, 2 ply, z-S twist
Average width: 0.13 cm
Passive elements: Cordage, 3 ply, z-S twist
Number of passive units: 24
Number in unit: 1 (except where doubled at toe)
Average width: 0.16 cm
Ties, loops, attachments: Toe: Cordage, ties 2 ply s-Z
　spun. Heel: Loops of 3 ply cordage Z twist (each
　ply 2 ply, z-S twist)
Shape: Left foot shaping, scalloped toe and
　puckered heel
Start: Scalloped toe start
Body: 2/2 alternate pair twining over doubled warps
　for forward one-third section of sandal at which
　point doubled warps end. Remaining 2/3 of
　sandal woven in raised geometric pattern
Finish: Puckered heel finish. Heel cords cross each
　other, stitch into sandal, loop, and stitch into
　sandal again.

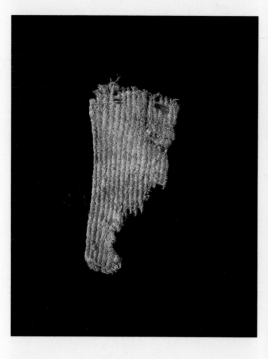

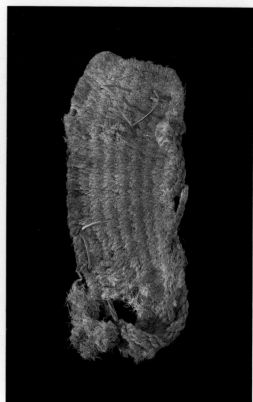

Catalog no.: 733.1
Site: Sega at Sosa (Tsegi Hatsosie) Canyon, Arizona
Collector and date: Byron Cummings, University of
    Utah Expedition, 1909
Cultural period: Basketmaker III (?)
Construction technique: Twined
Dimensions: Length 25.0 cm, width 10.2 cm, depth
    0.90 cm
Active elements: Cordage, 2 ply, z-S twist
Average width: 0.33 cm
Passive elements: Cordage, 2 ply, z-S twist
Number of passive units: 8-10(?)
Number in unit: 1
Average width: 0.27 cm
Ties, loops, attachments: Toe: Leaf element knotted
    on sole. Heel: Four strands of 2 ply, z-S twist are
    combined in Z twist to form a single heavy heel
    loop and one edge loop. These four strands
    appear to be extensions of the warp. Edge: Two
    edge loops, 2 ply, s-Z twist
Shape: Heart-shaped toe and puckered heel
Start: It appears that 4-5 elements fold at toe to
    form 8-10 warps. The outer warps appear to
    cross over each other; at center another warp
    folds, crossing the first two warps. Remaining
    warps fold inside the outer edge warp
Body: 1/1 simple twining from toe to heel
Finish: Puckered heel finish. Four warps emerge
    from each side after warps were pulled tightly to
    the center. One group is remnant but the other
    group emerges and loops along edge. This
    cordage is 4 ply, Z twist (each ply is 2 ply z-S
    twist).

144 Catalog no.: 3504.2
Site: Sega at Sosa (Tsegi Hatsosie) Canyon, Arizona
Collector and date: Byron Cummings, University of
    Utah Expedition, 1909
Cultural period: Basketmaker III
Construction technique: Composite
Dimensions: Length 14.5 cm, width 7.5 cm, depth
    0.46 cm
Active elements: Cordage, element 2 ply, z-S twist
Average width: 0.76 cm
Passive elements: Cordage, element 3 ply, z-S twist
Number of passive units: 16
Number in unit: 1
Average width: 0.11 cm
Ties, loops, attachments: Toe: Two stitches of coarse
    dark hair fiber. Heel: One stitch of yucca fiber.
Shape: Fragmentary
Start: Missing
Body: Twined forward section of sandal fragment.
    At heel there is approximately a 2 cm section
    that appears to be a wrapped weft section.
Finish: Most of heel is missing. On section that
    remains it appears warp ends are looped back
    into body of sandal.
Other: Sandal has been glued together.

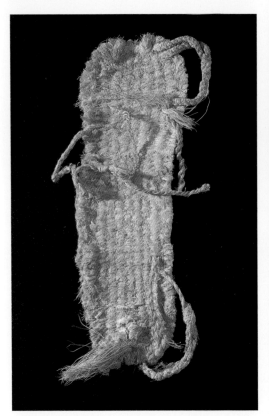

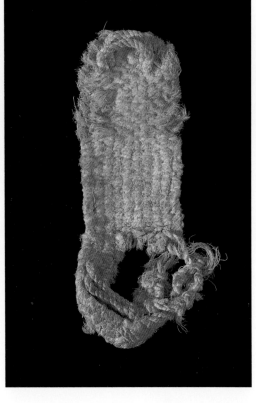

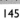

Catalog no.: 748

Site: Sega at Sosa (Tsegi Hatsosie) Canyon, Arizona

Collector and date: Byron Cummings, University of
Utah Expedition, 1909

Cultural period: Basketmaker III

Construction technique: Twined

Dimensions: Length 27.0 cm, width 9.0 cm, depth
1.0 cm

Active elements: Cordage, 2 ply, z-S twist

Average width: 0.35 cm

Passive elements: Cordage, 2 ply, z-S twist

Number of passive units: 10

Number in unit: 1

Average width: 0.35 cm

Ties, loops, attachments: Toe: Two remaining
separate cords on right side of toe, 2 ply, Z
twist (each ply 2 ply z-S twist)

Shape: Left(?) foot shaping, heart-shaped toe and
rounded heel

Start: It appears that 5 elements were folded at toe
to form 10 warps. The arrangement appears to
be that edge warps cross over each other at the
center; another element folds at center crossing
the first two warps; and two warps are folded
(one on each side) inside the outer edge warp.

Body: Sandal appears to be woven with 1/1 simple
twining for approximately 5-6 rows followed by a
row of three-element twining that creates a
ridge on the sole only.

Finish: Heel may have been puckered. Warps appear
wrapped around outer warp elements that have
been brought across to form heel cords.
Remaining heel cord 2 ply Z twist (each ply 2 ply
z-S twist)

Catalog no.: 731

Site: Sega at Sosa (Tsegi Hatsosie) Canyon, Arizona

Collector and date: Byron Cummings, University of
Utah Expedition, 1909

Cultural period: Basketmaker III (?)

Construction technique: Twined

Dimensions: Length 26.0 cm, width 8.8 cm, depth
0.82 cm

Active elements: Cordage, 2 ply, z-S twist

Passive elements: Cordage, 3 ply, z-S twist

Average width: 0.43 cm

Number of passive units: 10

Number in unit: 1 (except where doubled at toe)

Average width: 0.38 cm

Ties, loops, attachments: Toe: Two cordage loops, 3
ply, s-Z twist. Heel: Four cordage loops, 3 ply,
s-Z twist

Shape: Scalloped toe, puckered heel

Start: Scalloped toe start

Body: 2/2 twining(?) at toe over doubled toe warps.
1/1 simple twining for remaining two-thirds of
sandal

Finish: Puckered heel finish

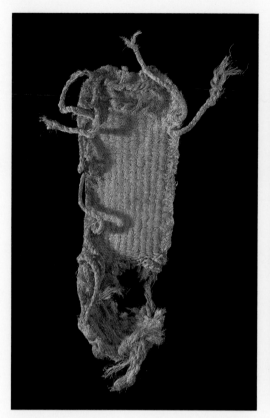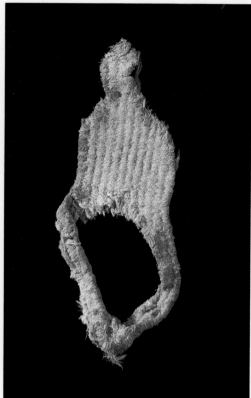

146 *Catalog no.:* 750

Site: Sega at Sosa (Tsegi Hatsosie) Canyon, Arizona

Collector and date: Byron Cummings, University of Utah Expedition, 1909

Cultural period: Basketmaker III(?)

Construction technique: Twined

Dimensions: Length 26.3 cm, width 8.8 cm, depth 0.56 cm

Active elements: Cordage, 2 ply, z-S twist

Average width: 0.19 cm

Passive elements: Cordage, 2 ply, z-S twist

Number of passive units: 14

Number in unit: 1 (except where doubled at toe)

Average width: 0.28 cm

Ties, loops, attachments: Toe: Two cordage loops, 3 ply, z-S twist. Heel: Loop emerges from knot of warps, 3 ply Z twist (each ply 2 ply z-S twist). Edge: Cordage loops, 2 ply Z twist (each ply 2 ply z-S twist). Cordage on left side looped and stitched into sandal

Shape: Scalloped toe and puckered heel

Start: Scalloped toe start, except twining is 1/1.

Body: Simple 1/1 twining at toe over doubled warps. Evidence of horizontal ridges spaced approximately 0.32 cm apart suggests several rows of simple twining and one row of three-element twining.

Finish: Puckered heel finish. Warp ends are turned back to upper surface where some are clipped short and the majority are gathered into a pair of thick knots. Heel loop emerges from largest knot.

Catalog no.: 766

Site: Sega at Sosa (Tsegi Hatsosie) Canyon, Arizona

Collector and date: Byron Cummings, University of Utah Expedition, 1909

Cultural period: Basketmaker III(?)

Construction technique: Twined

Dimensions: Length 25.0 cm, width 8.0 cm, depth 0.65 cm

Active elements: Cordage, 2 ply, z-S twist

Average width: 0.21 cm

Passive elements: Cordage, 2 ply, z-S twist

Number of passive units: 12

Number in unit: 1

Average width: 0.4 cm

Ties, loops, attachments: Heel: possible cord remnants

Shape: Toe missing, puckered heel

Start: Missing

Body: 2/2 alternate pair twining in fragment of toe area. The remainder of the sandal appears to be plain twining.

Finish: At heel warp, elements from both edges appear pulled and crossed at the heel. Evidence of remaining warp elements wrapping over heel cord

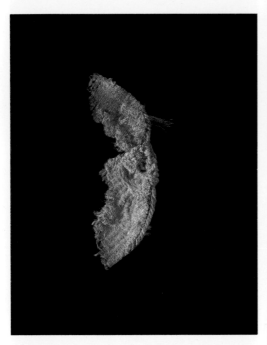

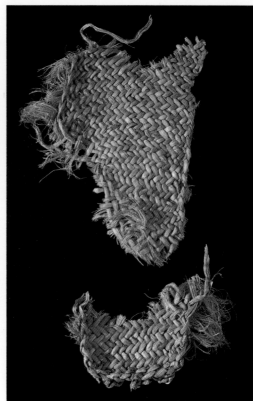

Catalog no.: 977
Site: Sega at Sosa (Tsegi Hatsosie) Canyon, Arizona
Collector and date: Byron Cummings, University of
    Utah Expedition, 1909
Cultural period: Basketmaker III(?)
Construction technique: Twined
Dimensions: Length 16.0 cm, width 6.8 cm, depth
    0.52 cm
Active elements: Cordage, 2 ply, z-S twist
Average width: 0.16 cm
Passive elements: Cordage, 3 ply, z-S twist
Number of passive units: 20
Number in unit: 1
Average width: 0.036 cm
Ties, loops, attachments: None apparent
Shape: Rounded toe, fragmentary
Start: Elements appear folded one inside the other
    at toe
Body: 1/1 plain twining for length of fragment
Finish: Missing

Catalog no.: 783.1 and 783.2
Site: Snake House, Arizona
Collector and date: Byron Cummings, University of
    Utah Expedition, 1909
Cultural period: Unknown
Construction technique: Plaited
Dimensions: No. 783.1, length 19.4 cm, width 11.0
    cm, depth 1.0 cm. No. 783.2, length 8.0 cm,
    width 8.0 cm, depth 11.0 cm
Active elements: Leaf element, unspun, cortex intact
Average width: 0.37 cm
Passive elements: N/A
Ties, loops, attachments: None apparent
Shape: Right foot shaping, rounded heel
Start: Missing
Body: 2/2 twill plaiting with shifts of 2/3/2 at selvage
    pulling tightly for shaping. Exhausted ends left
    frayed on sole
Finish: At heel ends appear looped around adjacent
    element and left protruding on sole.
Other: Structural padding on sole. Sandal is in two
    sections.

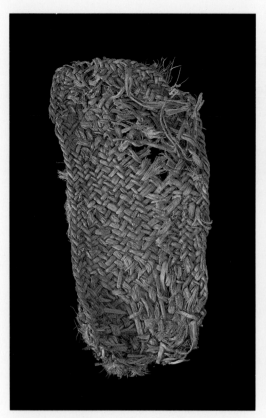
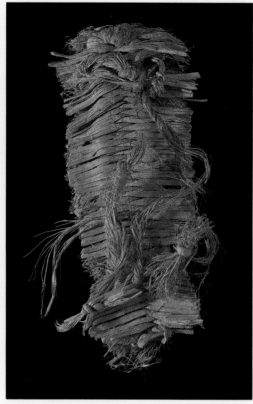

/ \\\ /// \\\ /// \\\ /// \\\ /// \\\ /// \\\ /// \\\ ///

148   *Catalog no.:* 7898
Site: Step Canyon, Arizona
Collector and date: Byron Cummings, University of
   Utah Expedition, 1926
Cultural period: Unknown
Construction technique: Plaited
Dimensions: Length 26.0 cm, width 13.0 cm, depth
   1.45 cm
Active elements: Leaf element unspun, cortex intact
Average width: 0.48 cm
Passive elements: N/A
Ties, loops, attachments: Toe and Edge: Leaf elements
   looped and stitched through sandal from middle
   of toe section to upper right edge
Shape: Right foot shaping, tapered toe with toe jog,
   rounded heel
Start: Active elements are folded at toe with
   additional elements added as toe tapers and
   forms a jog.
Body: 2/2 twill plaiting for length of sandal with
   shifts of 2/1/2. Edges are pulled in slightly.
   Exhausted ends left frayed on sole
Finish: Much of heel area is worn and patched but
   left side shows evidence of ends looped around
   adjacent elements and clipped short.
Other: Stitching using leaf element at heel and toe
   appears to be mends. Structural padding on sole

Catalog no.: 42KA274 (FS1) 23898
Site: Talus Ruin, Utah
Collector and date: UCRBSP, 1958
Cultural period: Pueblo II-Pueblo III
Construction technique: Plain weave
Dimensions: Length 26.00 cm, width 11.00 cm,
   depth 2.00 cm
Active elements: Leaf element unspun, cortex intact
Average width: 0.43 cm
Passive elements: Leaf element unspun, cortex intact
Number of passive units: 2
Number in unit: 1
Average width: 0.75 cm
Ties, loops, attachments: Toe: Two loops; one loop
   unspun leaf element and one loop S twist leaf
   element. Long tie of leaf element Z twist
   extends from toe to heel. Heel: Ankle loop S
   twist leaf element
Shape: Rounded toe and heel
Start: Two warps are tied together in one knot at
   toe.
Body: Over-under plain weave beginning with
   narrow ends of leaf element on top and ending
   with shredded wide ends on sole for padding.
   Ends extend beyond body of sandal.
Finish: At heel warps are tied together in a knot.
Other: Structural padding on sole

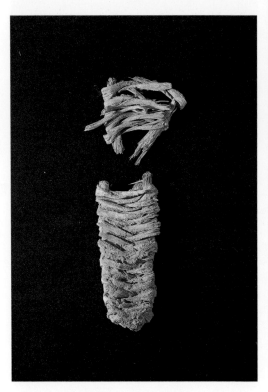

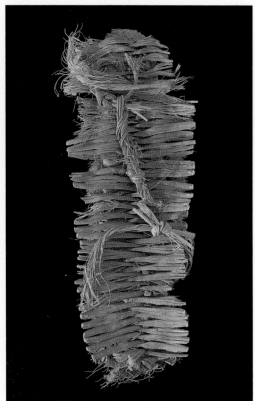

Catalog no.: 42KA274 (FS55.3) 23898
Site: Talus Ruin, Utah
Collector and date: UCRBASP, 1958
Cultural period: Pueblo II-Pueblo III
Construction technique: Plain weave
Dimensions: Two fragments: Length 12.50 cm, width 5.50 cm, depth 1.30 cm; Length 7.00 cm, width 6.50 cm, depth 0.70 cm
Active elements: Leaf element unspun, cortex intact
Average width: 0.70 cm
Passive elements: Leaf element unspun, cortex intact
Number of passive units: 2
Number in unit: 1
Average width: 0.79 cm
Ties, loops, attachments: None apparent
Shape: Rounded at end that is intact, but caked with mud
Start: It appears that warps are knotted at one end (narrowed point).
Body: Over-under plain weave beginning with narrow ends of leaf elements on top and ending with shredded, wide ends on sole for padding
Finish: Missing
Other: Structural padding on sole

Catalog no.: 42KA274 (FS101) 23898   149
Site: Talus Ruin, Utah
Collector and date: UCRBSP, 1958
Cultural period: Pueblo II-Pueblo III
Construction technique: Plain weave
Dimensions: Length 28.00 cm, width 11.00 cm, depth 3.90 cm
Active elements: Leaf element unspun, cortex intact
Average width: 0.56 cm
Passive elements: Leaf element unspun, cortex intact
Number of passive units: 2
Number in unit: 2 or 3?
Average width: 0.59 cm
Ties, loops, attachments: Toe: Leaf element loop, Z twist, stitched through body of sandal and knotted together at top with one square knot. Remnants of two cordage ties 2 ply, z-S twist extend from toe loop. One has a square knot. Heel: Leaf element S twist looped around body of sandal and secured on sole with shredded weft elements. One square knot at top
Shape: Rounded toe and heel
Start: Warps are tied in one knot at toe. Knot is wrapped.
Body: Over-under plain weave beginning with narrow ends of leaf element on top and ending with shredded wide ends on sole for padding. Ends extend beyond body of sandal.
Finish: At heel warps are tied together in two square knots stacked on top of each other.
Other: Structural padding on sole

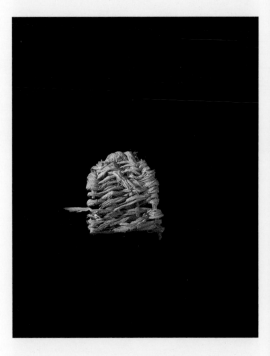

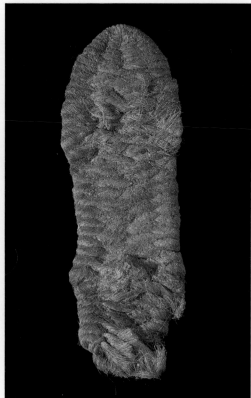

150 *Catalog no.:* 42GA288 (FS166.3) 24066
Site: Triangle Cave, Utah
Collector and date: UCRBASP, 1961
Cultural period: Pueblo II-Pueblo III
Construction technique: Plain weave
Dimensions: Length 6.5 cm, width 5.5 cm, depth 0.5
cm
Active elements: Leaf element unspun, cortex intact
Average width: 0.40 cm
Passive elements: Leaf element unspun, cortex intact
Number of passive units: 4
Number in unit: 1
Average width: 0.32 cm
Ties, loops, attachments: Possible loop fragment at
remaining end
Shape: Rounded toe, finish missing, fragmentary
Start: Warps are tied together in three knots at
toe. Weft stitches around knots.
Body: Over-under plain weave with shredded ends
left on sole for padding
Other: Structural padding on sole

Catalog no.: 1591.1
Site: Turkey House, Arizona
Collector and date: Byron Cummings, University of
Utah Expedition, 1911
Cultural period: Pueblo I-Pueblo II
Construction technique: Plain weave
Dimensions: Length 29.8 cm, width 10.4 cm, depth
1.2 cm
Active elements: Shredded leaf material, twisted S
and Z
Average width: 0.69 cm
Passive elements: Cordage, 2 ply, s-Z twist
Number of passive units: 4
Number in unit: 1
Average width: 0.36 cm
Ties, loops, attachments: Toe: 1 cordage tie, 2 ply,
s-Z twist
Shape: Pointed toe and squared heel
Start: Two cordage warps folded at toe (one inside
the other) to form four warps. Finer active
wefts used at start to draw in toe
Body: Tightly packed plain weave continues to heel.
Shredded yucca weft has been gathered together
for appropriate width of weft and twisted as it is
woven. This gives an "S" twist in one direction
and a "Z" twist in the opposite direction.
Finish: At heel it appears warps are woven back
into sandal.

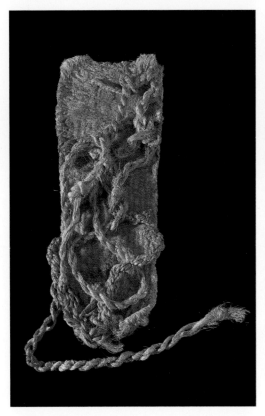
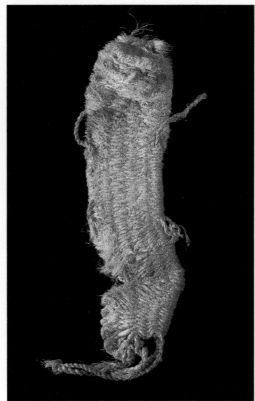

Catalog no.: 1592
Site: Turkey House, Arizona
Collector and date: Byron Cummings, University of
    Utah Expedition, 1911
Cultural period: Basketmaker III (?)
Construction technique: Plain weave and twined
Dimensions: Length 25.0 cm, width 10.0 cm, depth
    0.60 cm
Active elements: Cordage, 2 ply, z-S twist
Average width: 0.23 cm
Passive elements: Cordage, 2 ply, z-S twist
Number of passive units: 16
Number in unit: 1 (except where doubled at toe)
Average width: 0.34 cm
Ties, loops, attachments: Toe: One two-ply, z-S twist
    cord looped across middle toe area. Two large
    cords, 2 ply S twist (each ply 2 ply, s-Z twist)
    extend from right toe. One cord loop is sewn
    into side of sandal and is knotted to a long tie.
    Other cord laces through loops and tie end
    extends beyond length of sandal. Edge: Cords
    appear to be warps. Six warps extending from
    heel with 2 groups of three twisting together
    and sewn into sides of sandal
Shape: Some toe area missing but appears
    scalloped, puckered heel.
Start: Scalloped toe start
Body: 2/2 alternate pair twining over doubled warps
    at toe Instep to heel appears to be 3(?) rows
    plain weave and one row of 3 element twining
    creating a ridge on sole only. Heel area is very
    worn.
Finish: Puckered heel finish

Catalog no.: 1594.1
Site: Turkey House, Arizona
Collector and date: Byron Cummings, University of
    Utah Expedition, 1911
Cultural period: Pueblo I-Pueblo II
Construction technique: Plain weave
Dimensions: Length 27.0 cm, width 7.0 cm, depth
    0.9 cm
Active elements: Shredded leaf element, twisted S
    and Z
Average width: 0.20 cm
Passive elements: Cordage, 2 ply, s-Z twist
Number of passive units: 3
Number in unit: 1
Average width: 0.2 cm
Ties, loops, attachments: Toe: Leaf element remnant
    loops around a warp then twists back on itself.
    Edges: Cordage, 2 ply, s-Z twist. Heel: Six warps
    extend from end of sandal.
Shape: Rounded toe, heel disarticulating
Start: Three warps folded at toe (one inside the
    other) to form six warps. Finer active wefts used
    at start to draw in toe
Body: Tightly packed plain weave continues to heel.
    Shredded yucca weft has been gathered together
    for appropriate width of weft and twisted as it is
    woven. This gives an "S" twist in one direction
    and a "Z" twist in the opposite direction.
Finish: Unknown
Other: At toe a 3 cm long, four-warp woven piece
    in a round shape has been joined to top of
    sandal.

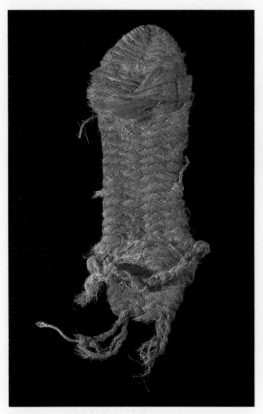 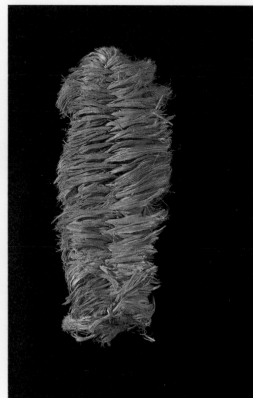

152 Catalog no.: 1596
Site: Turkey House, Arizona
Collector and date: Byron Cummings, University of
   Utah Expedition, 1911
Cultural period: Pueblo I-Pueblo II
Construction technique: Plain weave
Dimensions: Length 27.0 cm, width 11.0 cm, depth
   1.3 cm
Active elements: Shredded leaf material, twisted S
   and Z
Average width: 0.63 cm
Passive elements: Cordage, 3 ply, z-S twist
Number of passive units: 4
Number in unit: 1
Average width: 0.37 cm
Ties, loops, attachments: Heel: ankle loop 2 ply Z
   twist cordage (each ply 2 ply z-S twist). Hide
   wrapped on several areas of cord. Warps extend
   as ties from heel. Small cordage 2 ply, s-Z twist
   attached to left warp tie
Material: Yucca sp., hide
Shape: Left foot shaping, pointed toe, straight heel
Start: At toe two warps fold to make four warps.
   Weft begins plain weave interlacement at toe.
Body: Tightly packed plain weave continues to heel.
   Weft is shredded yucca that has been gathered
   together for appropriate width of weft and
   twisted as it is woven. This gives an "S" twist in
   one direction and a "Z" twist in the opposite
   direction.
Finish: At heel warps trail but were probably part
   of the tie system.
Other: Hide wrapped in some areas at ankle cord

Catalog no.: 1597.1
Site: Turkey House, Arizona
Collector and date: Byron Cummings, University of
   Utah Expedition, 1911
Cultural period: Pueblo II-Pueblo III
Construction technique: Plain weave
Dimensions: Length 22 cm, width 9 cm, depth 1.5
   cm
Active elements: Leaf element unspun, cortex intact
Average width: 0.4 cm
Passive elements: Leaf element unspun, cortex intact
Number of passive units: 2
Number in unit: 1
Average width: 0.67 cm
Ties, loops, attachments: None remaining
Shape: Pointed toe, rounded heel, with a narrowing
   at heel
Start: Two warps are tied together at toe in one
   knot.
Body: Over-under plain weave, beginning with
   narrow ends of leaf element on top and ending
   with shredded wide ends on sole for padding.
   Ends extend beyond body of sandal.
Finish: At heel warps are tied in three knots.
Other: Structural padding on sole

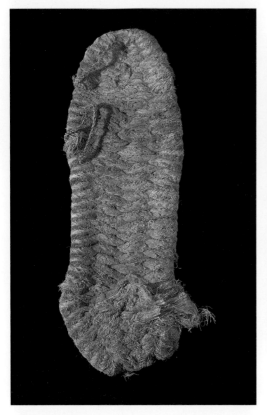

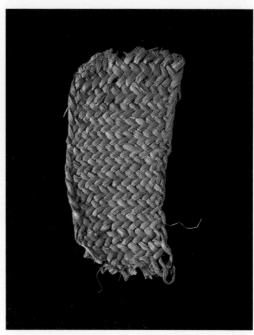

Catalog no.: 1598.1
Site: Turkey House, Arizona
Collector and date: Byron Cummings, University of
Utah Expedition, 1911
Cultural period: Pueblo I-Pueblo II
Construction technique: Plain weave
Dimensions: Length 26.8 cm, width 9.5 cm, depth
1.4 cm
Active elements: Shredded leaf element, twisted S
and Z
Average width: 0.66 cm
Passive elements: Cordage, 2 ply, s-Z twist
Number of passive units: 4
Number in unit: 1
Average width: 0.46 cm
Ties, loops, attachments: Edge: Two cordage loops; Z
twist, 2 ply (each ply, z-S twist)
Shape: Rounded toe and heel
Start: Two warps folded at toe (one inside the
other) to form four warps. Finer active weft
elements used at start to draw in toe
Body: Tightly packed plain weave continues to heel.
Shredded yucca weft has been gathered together
for appropriate width of weft and twisted as it is
woven. This gives an "S" twist in one direction
and a "Z" twist in the opposite direction.
Finish: At heel it appears warps are woven back
into sandal.

Catalog no.: 1599
Site: Turkey House, Arizona
Collector and date: Byron Cummings, University of
Utah Expedition, 1911
Cultural period: Pueblo II-Pueblo III
Construction technique: Plaited
Dimensions: Length 19.0 cm, width 9.50 cm, depth
0.69 cm
Active elements: Leaf element unspun, cortex intact
Average width: 0.50 cm
Passive elements: N/A
Ties, loops, attachments: None apparent
Shape: Left foot shaping, tapered toe, heel missing
Start: Twelve double elements are aligned parallel
and twined. These elements are then folded
double forming 24 active elements. Twining
visible on only one side after folding.
Body: 2/2 twill plaiting using doubled active
elements for approximately one-third when
doubled elements end and weaving is with single
elements. At edges elements turn back into the
weaving alternating upper side with sole.
Finish: Missing

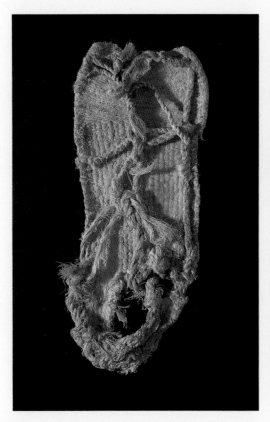
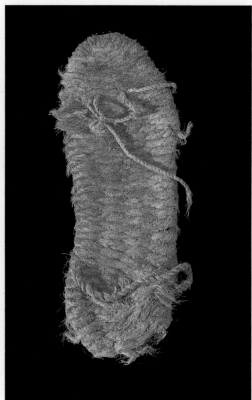

154 Catalog no.: 1601
Site: Turkey House, Arizona
Collector and date: Byron Cummings, University of
Utah Expedition, 1911
Cultural period: Basketmaker III (?)
Construction technique: Plain weave and twined
Dimensions: Length 26.0 cm, width 11.0 cm, depth
0.91 cm
Active elements: Cordage, 2 ply, z-S twist
Average width: 0.26 cm
Passive elements: Cordage, 2 ply, z-S twist
Number of passive units: 24
Number in unit: 1 (except where doubled at toe)
Average width: 0.35 cm
Ties, loops, attachments: Heel: Heavy cordage 2 ply
Z twist (formed from warps). Edge: Cordage, 2
ply, s-Z twist loops and stitches down both
edges. Some mending and knots. Lacing across
edge cords with 2 ply s-Z twist cordage
Shape: Scalloped toe and puckered heel
Start: Scalloped toe start
Body: 2/2 alternate pair twining over doubled warps
for toe section. Remainder of sandal appears to
be approximately three rows of plain weave and
one row of three element twining creating a
ridge on sole.
Finish: Puckered heel finish. Heel cords of warp are
twisted Z. They cross from each side and
connect with edge cords.

Catalog no.: 1602
Site: Turkey House, Arizona
Collector and date: Byron Cummings, University of
Utah Expedition, 1911
Cultural period: Pueblo I-Pueblo II
Construction technique: Plain weave
Dimensions: Length 26.5 cm, width 10.0 cm, depth
1.3 cm
Active elements: Shredded leaf material, twisted S
and Z
Average width: 0.54 cm
Passive elements: Cordage, 4 ply, Z twist (each ply
z-S twist)
Number of passive units: 4
Number in unit: 1
Average width: 0.54 cm
Ties, loops, attachments: Toe: Two loops and two
ties next to loops are cordage, 2 ply z-S twist.
Heel: Cordage, loop, 2 ply, z-S twist
Shape: Slightly shaped for right foot, pointed toe,
squared heel
Start: Two warps folded at toe one inside the other
to form four warps. Weft begins plain weave
interlacement at toe.
Body: Tightly packed plain weave continues to heel.
Weft is shredded yucca that has been gathered
together for appropriate width of weft and
twisted as it is woven. This gives an "S" twist in
one direction and a "Z" twist in the opposite
direction.
Finish: Disarticulating heel area prevents
determining finish.

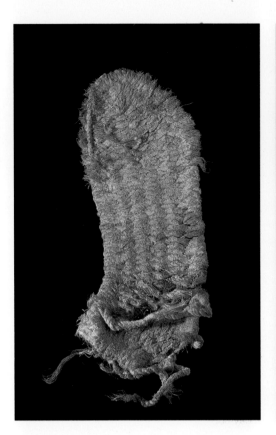

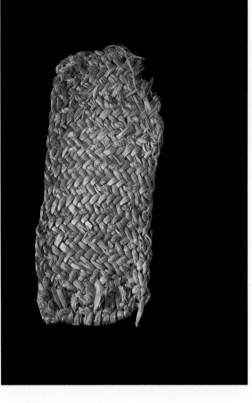

Catalog no.: 1603.1
Site: Turkey House, Arizona
Collector and date: Byron Cummings, University of
  Utah Expedition, 1911
Cultural period: Pueblo I-Pueblo II
Construction technique: Plain weave
Dimensions: Length 24 cm, width 10 cm, depth 0.8
  cm
Active elements: Shredded leaf element, twisted S
  and Z
Average width: 0.39 cm
Passive elements: Cordage, 2 ply, s-Z twist
Number of passive units: 6
Number in unit: 1
Average width: 0.35 cm
Ties, loops, attachments: Heel: Cordage (each ply 3
  ply, s-Z twist) looped and stitched through on
  each side of sandal, 2 ply, Z twist. Three cordage
  lacings at heel, 2 ply, s-Z twist. One heel lacing
  knotted to a heel warp
Shape: Right foot shaping, rounded toe and heel
Start: Three warps folded at toe (one inside the
  other) to form six warps. Finer wefts used at
  start to draw in toe
Body: Tightly packed plain weave continues to heel.
  Shredded yucca weft has been gathered together
  for appropriate width of weft and twisted as it is
  woven. This gives an "S" twist in one direction
  and a "Z" twist in the opposite direction.
Finish: Two broken ends of warps extend from heel
  area.

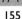

Catalog no.: 1612
Site: Turkey House, Utah
Collector and date: Byron Cummings, University of
  Utah Expedition, 1911
Cultural period: Pueblo II-Pueblo III
Construction technique: Plaited
Dimensions: Length 22.0 cm, width 9.5 cm, depth
  0.6 cm
Active elements: Leaf element unspun, cortex intact
Average width: 0.48 cm
Passive elements: N/A
Ties, loops, attachments: None appparent
Shape: Slightly rounded toe and squared heel
Start: Approximately 14 elements folded at toe to
  form 28 elements. Evidence of twined row of
  two ply cordage s-Z twist is incorporated
  immediately after the fold.
Body: 2/2 twill plaiting of single elements continues
  for the length of sandal.
Finish: It appears that an outer edge plaiting
  element has been extended across heel end and
  half of the elements have been brought over the
  top, wrapped around and brought to upper
  surface, then clipped. Alternating active elements
  are clipped short at heel on sole.
Other: Material added for padding. On the upper
  surface, 2 ply, s-Z twist cordage has been
  stitched across the sandal from side to side in
  parallel rows. This cordage attaches on the
  reverse side to a heavier braided cordage which
  runs in a continuum from side to side the length
  of sandal.

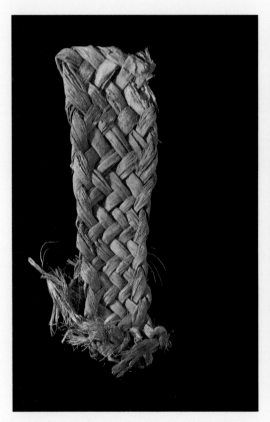

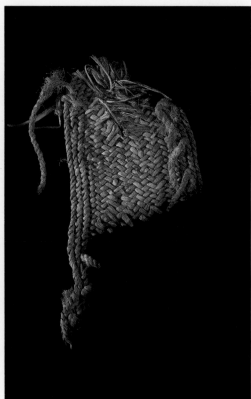

156 *Catalog no.:* 1613
Site: Turkey House, Arizona
Collector and date: Byron Cummings, University of
Utah Expedition, 1911
Cultural period: Pueblo II-Pueblo III
Construction technique: Plaited
Dimensions: Length 25.0 cm, width 8.0 cm, depth
1.0 cm
Active elements: Leaf element unspun, cortex intact
Average width: 1.2 cm
Passive elements: N/A
Ties, loops, attachments: One length of leaf element
attached to bottom of sandal near heel by a knot
Shape: Right foot shaping, squared toe and heel
Start: At toe five doubled elements are folded.
Body: 2/2 twill plaiting for length of sandal. Double
element plaiting from toe continuing about two-
thirds of sandal length; remaining one-third is
single element plaiting.
Finish: At heel, leaf element is folded across heel
forming two bars and secured at one end by a
knot. The plaiting elements are folded over these
bars in a pattern of every-other-one, the ends of
one group being brought to the surface, the
other to the reverse side.

Catalog no.: 1614
Site: Turkey House, Arizona
Collector and date: Byron Cummings, University of
Utah Expedition, 1911
Cultural period: Pueblo II-Pueblo III
Construction technique: Plaited
Dimensions: Length 23.0 cm, width 0.7 cm, depth
1.10 cm
Active elements: Leaf element unspun, cortex intact
Average width: 0.42 cm
Passive elements: N/A
Ties, loops, attachments: Edge: Cordage on both
sides, s-Z twist
Shape: Rounded toe partially missing, heel missing
Start: Missing
Body: 2/2 twill plaiting with three intervals on edges
pulled tightly creating three ridges. Exhausted
wide ends left frayed on sole
Finish: Missing
Other: Structural padding on sole. Mends on toe
and down body of sandal

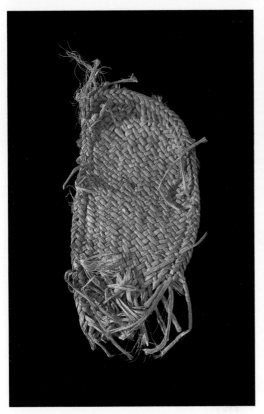
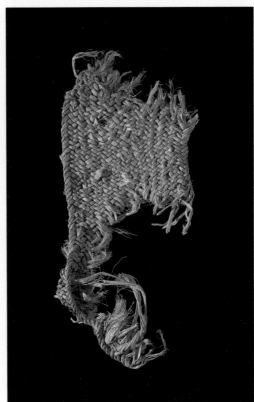

Catalog no.: 1616
Site: Turkey House, Arizona
Collector and date: Byron Cummings, University of
    Utah Expedition, 1911
Cultural period: Pueblo II-Pueblo III
Construction technique: Plaited
Dimensions: Length 22.7 cm, width 10.0 cm, depth
    0.79 cm
Active elements: Leaf element unspun, cortex intact
Average width: 0.34 cm
Passive elements: N/A
Ties, loops, attachments: Toe: Remnants of leaf
    element ties protrude. Edge: Leaf element ties
    knotted to sole
Shape: Right foot shaping, round tapered toe, heel
    missing
Start: Active elements folded at toe to begin one
    edge. Elements are spliced in to form a second
    edge. Short distance from start layers merge and
    2/2 twill plaiting continues on one layer. Shifts of
    2/3/2 occur for shaping. Exhausted wide ends
    left frayed on sole
Finish: Missing
Other: Structural padding on sole

Catalog no.: 1617
Site: Turkey House, Arizona
Collector and date: Byron Cummings, University of
    Utah Expedition, 1911
Cultural period: Pueblo II-Pueblo III
Construction technique: Plaited
Dimensions: Length 24.0 cm, width 11.0 cm, depth
    0.51 cm
Active elements: Leaf element unspun, cortex intact
Average width: 0.34 cm
Passive elements: N/A
Ties, loops, attachments: Heel: Leaf element loop
    twisted S
Shape: Left foot shaping, toe jog, heel missing
Start: Missing
Body: 2/2 twill plaiting with 2/1/2 shift for shaping,
    and 2/3/2 on edges which are pulled tight.
    Exhausted ends left frayed on sole
Finish: It appears alternate ends were wrapped with
    ends left protruding.
Other: Structural padding on sole

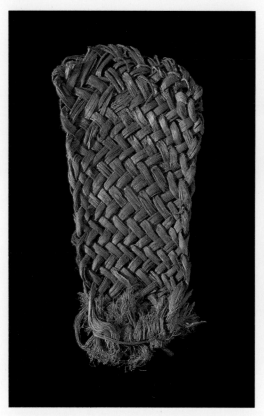

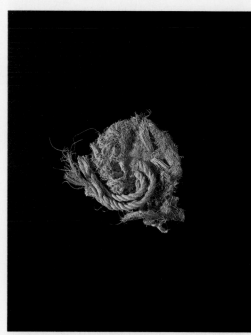

158 *Catalog no.:* 1618
Site: Turkey House, Arizona
Collector and date: Byron Cummings, University of
Utah Expedition, 1911
Cultural period: Pueblo II-Pueblo III
Construction technique: Plaited
Dimensions: Length 25.0 cm, width 12.0 cm, depth
0.8 cm
Active elements: Leaf element unspun, cortex intact
Average width: 0.65 cm
Passive elements: N/A
Ties, loops, attachments: Remnants of ties on both
surfaces
Shape: Right foot shaping, squared heel, rounded
toe
Start: Ten single elements folded to form 20
elements at toe; secured with twining near top
of toe edge. Knot at one end of twining
Body: 2/2 twill plaiting for length of sandal. Several
elements appear to have been dropped about
half-way down for shaping. Edges pulled in to
create a ridge
Finish: Leaf element folded across heel forming two
bars and secured at one end by a knot. The
plaiting elements are folded over the bar in a
pattern of every-other-one, the ends of one
group being brought to the upper surface side,
the others to the reverse side. All ends are
clipped.

Catalog no.: 1621.1
Site: Turkey House, Arizona
Collector and date: Byron Cummings, University of
Utah Expedition, 1911
Cultural period: Pueblo I-Pueblo II
Construction technique: Plain weave
Dimensions: Length 8 cm, width 7 cm, depth 0.9 cm
Active elements: Shredded leaf element, twisted S
and Z
Average width: 0.29 cm
Passive element: Cordage, 3 ply, z-S twist
Number of passive units: 6
Number in unit: 1
Average width: 0.5 cm
Ties, loops, attachments: Three ties, 3 ply, s-Z twist,
extend from center of fragment.
Shape: Rounded toe(?), missing heel, fragmentary
Start: Three warps folded at toe (one inside the
other) to form six warps
Body: Tightly packed plain weave. Shredded yucca
weft has been gathered together for appropriate
width of weft and twisted as it is woven. This
gives an "S" twist in one direction and a "Z"
twist in the opposite direction.
Finish: Missing
Other: Piece of corticated leaf element inserted
through sandal, with two ends visible on obverse
side

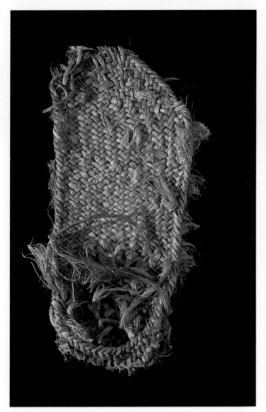 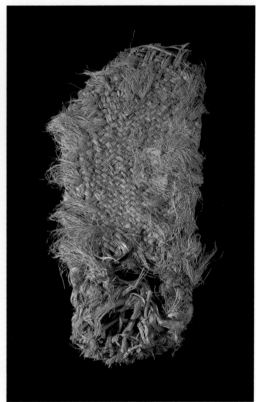

Catalog no.: 1620
Site: Turkey House, Arizona
Collector and date: Byron Cummings, University of
   Utah Expedition, 1911
Cultural period: Pueblo II-Pueblo III
Construction technique: Plaited
Dimensions: Length 25.5 cm, width 11.4 cm, depth
   0.81 cm
Active elements: Leaf element unspun, cortex intact
Average width: 0.39 cm
Passive elements: N/A
Ties, loops, attachments: Heel: Leaf element ties of Z
   twist are loose. Edge: Knot on right side
Shape: Right foot shaping, round tapered toe with
   toe jog, round cupped heel
Start: Approximately 10 elements folded at toe to
   form 20 active elements. One additional element
   folded for toe jog
Body: 2/2 twill plaiting for length of sandal. Edges
   plaited 2/3/2 and pulled in tight at heel.
   Exhausted ends left frayed on sole
Finish: At heel ends appear looped back into sandal.
Other: Structural padding on sole. Mends at heel
   and stitches in toe area

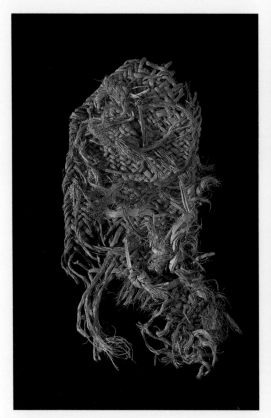

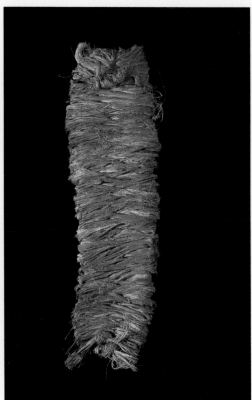

160 *Catalog no.:* 1622
Site: Turkey House, Arizona
Collector and date: Byron Cummings, University of
Utah Expedition, 1911
Cultural period: Pueblo II-Pueblo III
Construction technique: Plaited
Dimensions: Length 25.0 cm, width 11.0 cm, depth
0.50 cm
Active elements: Leaf element unspun, cortex intact
Average width: 0.46 cm
Passive elements: N/A
Ties, loops, attachments: Toe: Leaf element tie on left
side knotted to edge loops. Lacings of 2 ply s-Z
twist cordage and leaf elements. Edge, lacing of
leaf elements knotted together. Heel: Near heel
leaf element knotted
Shape: Left foot shaping, tapered toe with toe jog,
heel missing
Start: Active elements folded at toe. One folded
element is added for toe jog.
Body: 2/2 twill plaiting with shifts of 2/1/2 for
shaping and 2/3/2 on edges which are pulled
tight. Exhausted ends left frayed on sole
Finish: Missing
Other: Structural padding on sole

Catalog no.: 1623.1
Site: Turkey House, Arizona
Collector and date: Byron Cummings, University of
Utah Expedition, 1911
Cultural period: Pueblo II-Pueblo III
Construction technique: Plain weave
Dimensions: Length 24.5 cm, width 7.5 cm, depth
1.2 cm
Active elements: Leaf element unspun, cortex intact
Average width: 0.48 cm
Passive elements: Leaf element unspun, cortex intact
Number of passive units: 2
Number in unit: 1
Average width: 1.0 cm
Ties, loops, attachments: Toe: Shredded leaf element
loop, twisted S, attached to leaf element, cortex
intact, and knotted with narrow leaf element
Shape: Rounded toe and squared heel
Start: Two warps are tied together at toe in one
knot.
Body: Over-under plain weave with long wefts
encircling warps tightly ending with shredded
ends on sole for padding
Finish: At heel, each warp has been split and the
resulting 4 elements are tied in 2 contiguous
knots.

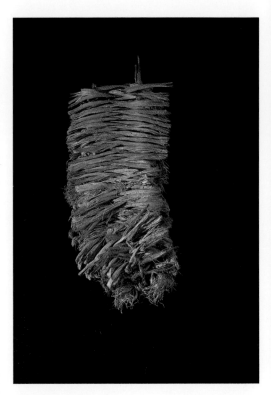
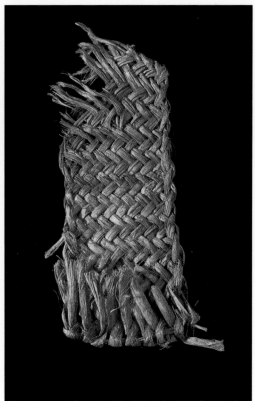

Catalog no.: 1624.1
Site: Turkey House, Arizona
Collector and date: Byron Cummings, University of
 Utah Expedition, 1911
Cultural period: Pueblo II-Pueblo III
Construction technique: Plain weave
Dimensions: Length 20.0 cm, width 8.5 cm, depth
 1.8 cm
Active elements: Leaf element unspun, cortex intact
Average width: 0.4 cm
Passive elements: Leaf element unspun, cortex intact
Number of passive units: 2
Number in unit: 1
Average width: 0.60 cm
Ties, loops, attachments: None apparent
Shape: Rounded toe, fragmentary
Start: Warps are tied together in two knots at toe.
Body: Over-under plain weave beginning with
 narrow ends of leaves on top and ending with
 shredded wide ends on sole for padding. Ends
 extend beyond body of sandal.
Finish: Missing
Other: Carbonization

Catalog no.: 1625
Site: Turkey House, Arizona
Collector and date: Byron Cummings, University of
 Utah Expedition, 1911
Cultural period: Pueblo II-Pueblo III
Construction technique: Plaited
Dimensions: Length 26.0 cm, width 10.0 cm, depth
 0.6 cm
Active elements: Leaf element unspun, cortex intact
Average width: 0.5 cm
Passive elements: N/A
Ties, loops, attachments: None
Shape: Squared toe and heel
Start: Single elements folded at toe. Disarticulation
 at one edge
Body: 2/2 twill plaiting for length of sandal
Finish: Leaf element folded across heel forming a
 doubled bar. The plaiting elements are folded
 over these two bars in a pattern of every-other-
 one, the ends of one group being brought to the
 upper surface, the others to the reverse side.

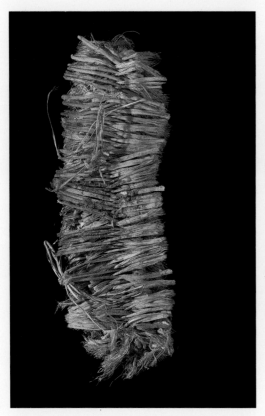

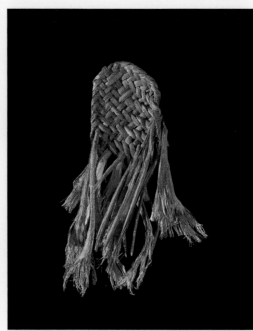

162 *Catalog no.:* 1646.1
Site: Turkey House, Arizona
Collector and date: Byron Cummings, University of
  Utah Expedition, 1911
Cultural period: Pueblo II-Pueblo III
Construction technique: Plain weave
Dimensions: Length 27.0 cm, width 9.1 cm, depth
  2.6 cm
Active elements: Leaf element unspun, cortex intact
Average width: 0.4 cm
Passive elements: Leaf element unspun, cortex intact
Number of passive units: 2
Number in unit: 3
Average width: 0.68 cm
Ties, loops, attachments: Toe: Loop of separated leaf
  element, cortex intact. Heel: Loop of separated
  leaf element, cortex intact
Shape: Left foot shaping(?), rounded toe and heel
Start: Two warps are tied together at toe in one
  knot.
Body: Over-under plain weave beginning with
  narrow ends of leaves on top and ending with
  shredded wide ends on sole for padding. Short
  wefts encircle warps tightly, beginning and ending
  beyond warp edge.
Finish: At heel, warp ends culminate in two knots.

Catalog no.: 1648
Site: Turkey House, Arizona
Collector and date: Byron Cummings, University of
  Utah Expedition, 1911
Cultural period: Pueblo II-Pueblo III
Construction technique: Plaited
Dimensions: Length 18.50 cm, width 6.50 cm, depth
  0.56 cm
Active elements: Leaf element unspun, cortex intact
Average width: 0.41 cm
Passive elements: N/A
Ties, loops, attachments: None apparent
Shape: Rounded toe.
Start: Eleven elements are folded at toe to form 22
  active elements.
Body: 2/2 twill plaiting with a 1/3 shift at beginning,
  a 1/3/1/3 shift at the center and a 2/1/2 shift
  near end of weaving
Finish: Unknown, sandal incomplete

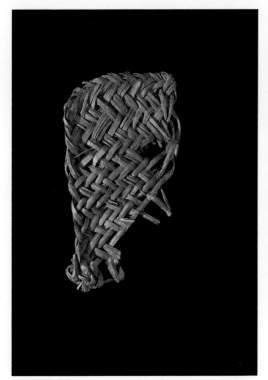

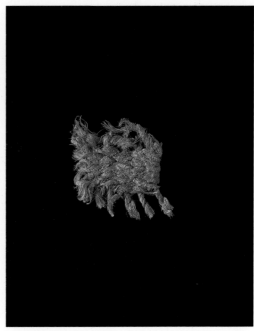

Catalog no.: 1693.1

Site: Turkey House, Arizona

Collector and date: Byron Cummings, University of
Utah Expedition, 1911

Cultural period: Pueblo II-Pueblo III

Construction technique: Plaited

Dimensions: Length 16.5 cm, width 9.5 cm, depth
0.7 cm

Active elements: Leaf element unspun, cortex intact

Average width: 0.45 cm

Passive elements: N/A

Ties, loops, attachments: None apparent

Shape: Left foot shaping

Start: Eight doubled elements, side by side, folded
to form 16 elements

Body: 2/2 twill plaiting for length of sandal

Finish: Missing except for one corner where a leaf
element folds at the side to form two bars over
which the plaiting elements fold and are carried
to the upper surface or reverse sides in an
every-other-one pattern

Catalog no.: 1694.1

Site: Turkey House, Arizona

Collector and date: Byron Cummings, University of
Utah Expedition, 1911

Cultural period: Pueblo I-Pueblo II

Construction technique: Plain weave

Dimensions: Length 7.0 cm, width 7.0 cm, depth 0.8
cm

Active elements: Separated leaf element, twisted S
and Z

Average width: 0.44 cm

Passive elements: Cordage, 2 ply, s-Z twist

Number of passive units: 5(?)

Number in unit: 1

Average width: 0.37 cm

Ties, loops, attachments: None apparent

Shape: Fragment

Start: Missing

Body: Tightly packed plain weave. Shredded yucca
weft has been gathered together for appropriate
width of weft and twisted as it is woven. This
gives an "S" twist in one direction and a "Z"
twist in the opposite direction.

Finish: Missing

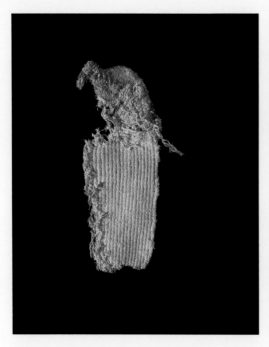
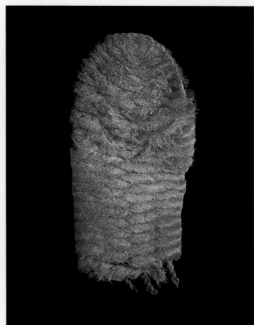

Catalog no.: 5002
Site: Turkey House, Arizona
Collector and date: Byron Cummings, University of
Utah Expedition, 1911
Cultural period: Pueblo I-Pueblo II
Construction technique: Plain weave
Dimensions: Length 21.30 cm, width 10.5 cm, depth
1.63 cm
Active elements: Shredded leaf element, twisted S
and Z
Average width: 0.81 cm
Passive elements: Cordage, 2 ply s-Z twist (each ply
is 2 ply z-S twist)
Number of passive units: 4
Number in unit: 1
Average width: 0.44 cm
Ties, loops, attachments: None apparent
Shape: Rounded toe, heel missing
Start: Two warps folded at toe (one inside the
other) to form four warps. Finer active wefts
used at start to draw into pointed toe shape
Body: Tightly packed plain weave continues to heel.
Shredded yucca weft has been gathered together
for appropriate width of weft and twisted as it is
woven. This gives an "S" twist in one direction
and a "Z" twist in the opposite direction.
Finish: Missing
Other: Charred

164   Catalog no.: 1695
Site: Turkey House, Arizona
Collector and date: Byron Cummings, University of
Utah Expedition, 1909
Cultural period: Basketmaker III
Construction technique: Composite
Dimensions: Length 16.8 cm, width 6.4 cm, depth
0.50 cm
Active elements: Cordage, 2 ply, z-S twist
Average width: 0.07 cm
Passive elements: Cordage, 3 ply, z-S twist
Number of passive units: 30
Number in unit: 1 (except where doubled at toe)
Average width: 0.32 cm
Ties, loops, attachments: Possible remnants
Shape: Scalloped toe, heel missing
Start: Scalloped toe start
Body: 2/2 alternate pair twining over doubled warps
for forward one-third section of sandal at which
point doubled warps end. There appears to be a
section of twining over single elements and then
a midsection of a knotted structure. Remaining
length of sandal to heel woven in raised
geometric pattern
Finish: Missing

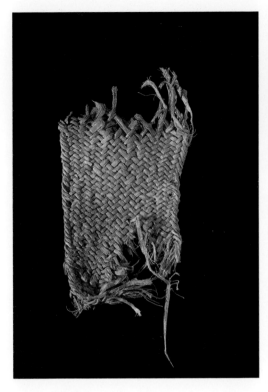
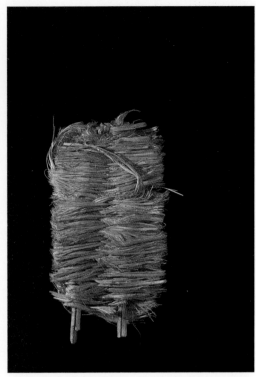

Catalog no.: 5003
Site: Turkey House, Arizona
Collector and date: Byron Cummings, University of
  Utah Expedition, 1911
Cultural period: Pueblo II-Pueblo III
Construction technique: Plaited
Dimensions: Length 15.16 cm, width 10.46 cm,
  depth 0.90 cm
Active elements: Leaf element unspun, cortex intact
Average width: 0.32 cm
Passive elements: N/A
Ties, loops, attachments: Possible awl holes along
  edges.
Shape: Cupped heel(?), toe missing
Start: Missing
Body: 2/2 twill plaiting with shifts of 2/3/2 in center
  for shaping and along edges which are pulled
  tight. Exhausted ends left frayed on sole
Finish: At heel plaiting pulled tight to draw up. Most
  of heel missing
Other: Structural padding on sole

Catalog no.: 5004
Site: Turkey House, Arizona
Collector and date: Byron Cummings, University of
  Utah Expedition, 1909
Cultural period: Pueblo II-Pueblo III
Construction technique: Plain weave
Dimensions: Length 16.5 cm, width 9.5 cm, depth
  1.6 cm
Active elements: Leaf element unspun, cortex intact
Average width: 0.28 cm
Passive elements: Leaf element unspun, cortex intact
Number of passive units: 2
Number in unit: 2
Average width: 0.70 cm
Ties, loops, attachments: Remnant of a loop passing
  around sandal
Shape: Squared heel, toe missing
Start: Missing
Body: Over-under plain weave beginning with
  narrow ends of leaf element on top and ending
  with shredded wide ends on sole for padding.
  Wefts encircle warps tightly, but ends extend
  beyond body of sandal
Finish: Heel finished with warps knotted together
  with two knots, one above the other
Other: Structural padding on sole

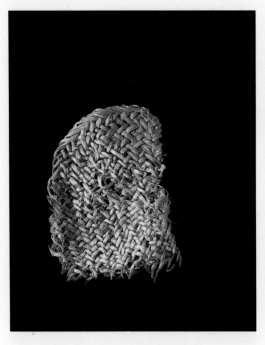 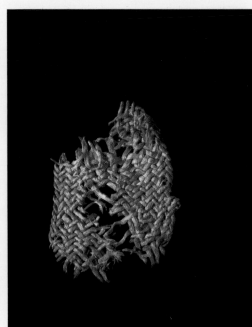

166 *Catalog no.:* 5005
Site: Turkey House, Arizona
Collector and date: Byron Cummings, University of
Utah Expedition, 1911
Cultural period: Pueblo II-Pueblo III
Construction technique: Plaited
Dimensions: Length 12.81 cm, width 9.13 cm, depth
0.30 cm
Active elements: Leaf element unspun, cortex intact
Average width: 0.27 cm
Passive elements: N/A
Ties, loops, attachments: None apparent
Shape: Left foot shaping, round tapered toe, heel
missing
Start: Active elements folded at toe
Body: 2/2 twill plaiting with some probable shifts in
center. 2/3/2 shift at edges. Exhausted wide ends
frayed on sole
Finish: Missing
Other: Structural padding on sole

Catalog no.: 5006
Site: Turkey House, Arizona
Collector and date: Byron Cummings, University of
Utah Expedition, 1911
Cultural period: Pueblo II-Pueblo III
Construction technique: Plaited
Dimensions: Length 13.5 cm, width 10.0 cm, depth
0.67 cm
Active elements: Leaf element unspun, cortex intact
Average width: 0.33 cm
Passive elements: N/A
Ties, loops, attachments: Toe: Small leaf element is
knotted on toe edge.
Shape: Right foot shaping, toe jog, fragmentary
Start: Missing
Body: 2/2 twill plaiting for length of fragment
Finish: Missing

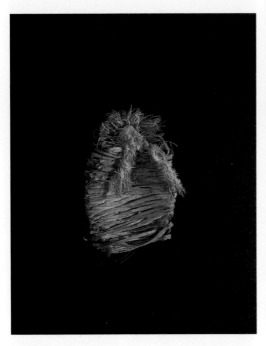

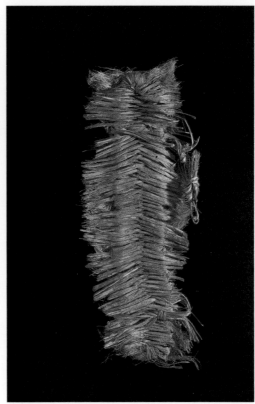

Catalog no.: AR3932 2843
Site: Turkey House, Arizona
Collector and date: Byron Cummings, University of
   Utah Expedition, 1911
Cultural period: Pueblo II-Pueblo III
Construction technique: Plain weave
Dimensions: Length 11.5 cm, width 7.5 cm, depth
   1.38 cm
Active elements: Leaf element unspun, cortex intact
Average width: 0.33 cm
Passive elements: Cordage, 2 ply, s-Z twist
Number of passive units: 2
Number in unit: 1
Average width: 0.42 cm
Ties, loops, attachments: Tie around warps of
   cordage 3(?) ply, s-Z twist
Shape: Rounded finished end
Start or Finish: Warps are tied together in one knot
   at toe.
Body: Over-under plain weave beginning with
   narrow ends of leaf element on top and ending
   with shredded wide ends on sole for padding
Other: Charred. Structural padding on sole

Catalog no.: 1711
Site: Twin Cave House, Arizona
Collector and date: Byron Cummings, University of
   Utah Expedition, 1913
Cultural period: Unknown
Construction technique: Plain weave
Dimensions: Length 28.5 cm, width 9.3 cm, depth
   1.4 cm
Active elements: Leaf element unspun, cortex intact
Average width: 0.29 cm
Passive elements: Leaf element unspun, cortex intact
Number of passive units: 2
Number in unit: 1
Average width: 0.58 cm
Ties, loops, attachments: Toe: Leaf element loops
   around toe. Another leaf element is tied to toe
   loop and knotted. Heel: Leaf element loops
   around heel and is knotted.
Shape: Rounded toe and heel
Start: Warps are tied together at toe in one knot.
Body: Over-under plain weave beginning with
   narrow ends of leaf element on top and ending
   with shredded wide ends on sole for padding.
   Wefts encircle warps both tightly and loosely
   which extends the width of sandal beyond the
   warp edge.
Finish: At heel warps are tied together in one knot.
Other: Structural padding on sole

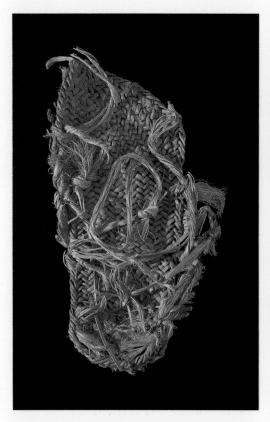 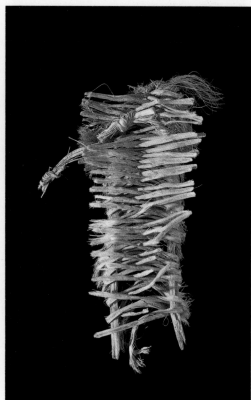

Catalog no.: 2821
Site: Twin Cave House, Arizona
Collector and date: Byron Cummings, University of
    Utah Expedition, 1913
Cultural period: Unknown
Construction technique: Plain weave
Dimensions: Length 21.0 cm, width 13.2 cm, depth
    0.75 cm
Active elements: Leaf element unspun, cortex intact
Average width: 0.43 cm
Passive elements: Leaf element unspun, cortex intact
Number of passive units: 2
Number in unit: 2
Average width: 0.71 cm
Ties, loops, attachments: Toe: Leaf element looped
    around toe and tied in a knot. Loose knotted tie
    on left side
Shape: Round toe, heel missing
Start: Warps are tied together at toe in one knot.
Body: Over-under plain weave beginning with
    narrow ends of leaf element on top and ending
    with shredded wide ends on sole for padding.
    Wefts encircle warps both tightly and loosely
    which extends the width of sandal beyond the
    warp edge.
Finish: Missing
Other: Structural padding on sole

168 Catalog no.: 2813
Site: Twin Cave House, Arizona
Collector and date: Byron Cummings, University of
    Utah Expedition, 1913
Cultural period: Pueblo II-Pueblo III
Construction technique: Plaited
Dimensions: Length 23.0 cm, width 10.5 cm, depth
    0.50 cm
Active elements: Leaf element, unspun, cortex intact
Average width: 0.44 cm
Passive elements: N/A
Ties, loops, attachments: Edge: Leaf element ties spun
    S begin at each side of toe, loop, and stitch
    down both sides and across heel. Additional leaf
    elements with a slight twist lace loop together.
Shape: Right foot shaping, tapered toe and round
    cupped heel
Start: Active elements fold at toe. Elements are
    added as needed for tapering.
Body: 2/2 twill plaiting for body of sandal. Shifts at
    toe to create shaping are variants of 2/2/1/2/2
    and 2/1/3/2/2. Edges pulled in 2/3/2 shift
Finish: At heel double edge pulled tight to create
    cupped heel
Other: Structural padding on heel

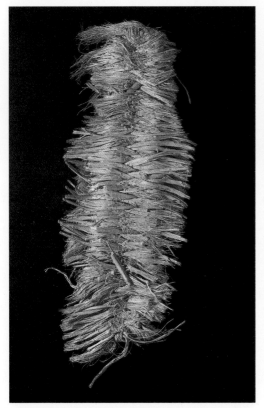
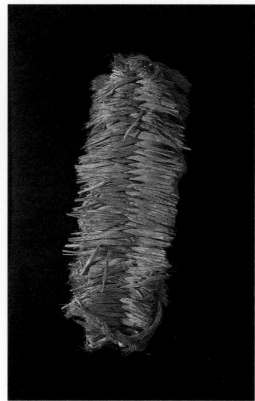

Catalog no.: 2822
Site: Twin Cave House, Arizona
Collector and date: Byron Cummings, University of
Utah Expedition, 1913
Cultural period: Unknown
Construction technique: Plain weave
Dimensions: Length 27.0 cm, width 10.5 cm, depth
1.1 cm
Active elements: Leaf element unspun, cortex intact
Average width: 0.38 cm
Passive elements: Leaf element unspun, cortex intact
Number of passive units: 2
Number in unit: 3
Average width: 0.60 cm
Ties, loops, attachments: Heel: Near heel a leaf
element encloses 3 or 4 wefts on a diagonal and
appears to protrude on sole.
Shape: Rounded toe and heel
Start: Warps are tied together at toe in one knot.
Body: Over-under plain weave beginning with
narrow ends of leaf element on top and ending
with shredded wide ends on sole for padding.
Ends extend beyond body of sandal, increasing
width.
Finish: At heel warp ends tied in two knots
Other: Structural padding on sole

Catalog no.: 2823
Site: Twin Cave House, Arizona
Collector and date: Byron Cummings, University of
Utah Expedition, 1913
Cultural period: Unknown
Construction technique: Plain weave
Dimensions: Length 23.5 cm, width 9.0 cm, depth
1.65 cm
Active elements: Leaf element unspun, cortex intact
Average width: 0.55 cm
Passive elements: Leaf element unspun, cortex intact
Number of passive units: 1
Number in unit: 1 or 2
Average width: 0.59 cm
Ties, loops, attachments: Heel: Two leaf element ties
extend from each side of heel and are knotted
together.
Shape: Rounded toe and heel
Start: Warps are tied together at toe in two knots.
Body: Over-under plain weave beginning with
narrow ends of leaf element on top and ending
with shredded wide ends on sole for padding.
Ends extend beyond body of sandal, increasing
width.
Finish: At heel warps are tied in two knots.
Other: Structural padding on sole

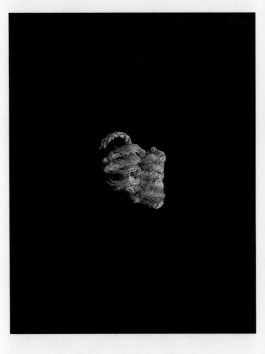
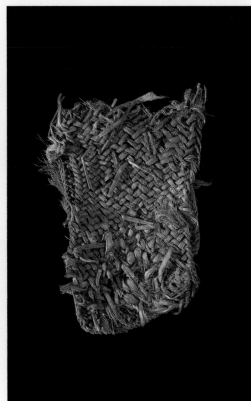

170   Catalog no.: 2824
       Site: Twin Cave House, Arizona
       Collector and date: Byron Cummings, University of
          Utah Expedition, 1913
       Cultural period: Pueblo I-Pueblo II
       Construction technique: Plain weave
       Dimensions: Length 6.6 cm, width 5.5 cm, depth
          1.25 cm
       Active elements: Shredded leaf elements, twisted S
          and Z
       Average width: 0.58 cm
       Passive elements: Cordage, 3 ply, s-Z twist
       Number of passive units: 2(?)
       Number in unit: 1
       Average width: 0.38 cm
       Ties, loops, attachments: None apparent
       Shape: Unknown, fragmentary piece
       Start: Unknown
       Body: Tightly packed plain weave continues to heel.
          Shredded yucca weft has been gathered together
          for appropriate width of weft and twisted as it is
          woven. This gives an "S" twist in one direction
          and a "Z" twist in the opposite direction.
       Finish: Unknown

Catalog no.: 2827
Site: Twin Cave House, Arizona
Collector and date: Byron Cummings, University of
   Utah Expedition, 1913
Cultural period: Pueblo II-Pueblo III
Construction technique: Plaited
Dimensions: Length 17.5 cm, width 11.0 cm, depth
   1.4 cm
Active elements: Leaf element unspun, cortex intact
Average width: Top: 0.35 cm Bottom: 0.24 cm
Passive elements: N/A
Ties, loops, attachments: Loose ties
Shape: Bottom layer has left foot shaping, tapered
   toe with jog. Top layer missing toe and heel
Start: It appears active elements were folded at toe
   for bottom layer, with elements folded and
   added for tapering and toe jog.
Body: 2/2 twill plaiting with shifts of 2/3/2 at edges
   on bottom layer. Exhausted ends left frayed on
   sole
Finish: Missing
Other: Structural padding on heel. Two fragmentary
   sandals stitched together with a leaf element

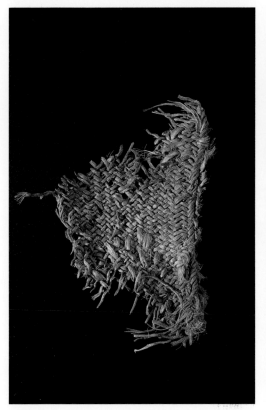
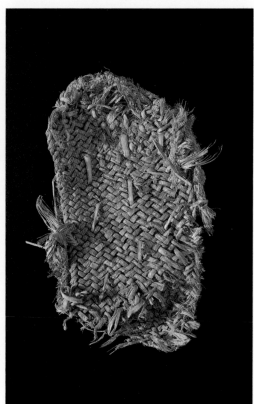

Catalog no.: 2829
Site: Twin Cave House, Arizona
Collector and date: Byron Cummings, University of
   Utah Expedition, 1913
Cultural period: Pueblo II-Pueblo III
Construction technique: Plaited
Dimensions: Length 19.0 cm, width 11.0 cm, depth
   0.62 cm
Active elements: Leaf element, unspun, cortex intact
Average width: 0.32 cm
Passive elements: N/A
Ties, loops, attachments: None apparent except one
   knot
Shape: Unknown, toe and heel missing, fragmentary
Start and Finish: Missing
Body: 2/2 twill plaiting for length of fragment. Shift
   of 2/3/2 on selvages. Piece appears narrowed
   toward heel. Exhausted ends frayed on sole
Other: Structural padding on sole

Catalog no.: 2830
Site: Twin Cave House, Arizona
Collector and date: Byron Cummings, University of
   Utah Expedition, 1913
Cultural period: Pueblo II-Pueblo III
Construction technique: Plaited
Dimensions: Length 22.0 cm, width 12.0 cm, depth
   1.40 cm
Active elements: Leaf element, unspun, cortex intact
Average width: Top: 0.36 cm Bottom: 0.28 cm
Passive elements: N/A
Ties, loops, attachments: Edge: Remnants of two
   loops on top sandal. Four knots along one edge.
   One loop remnant on bottom sandal
Shape: Unknown, toe and heel missing
Start and Finish: Missing
Body: 2/2 twill plaiting on both layers of joined
   sandals
Other: Two sandals bound together by three or
   four rows of running stitches from toe to heel

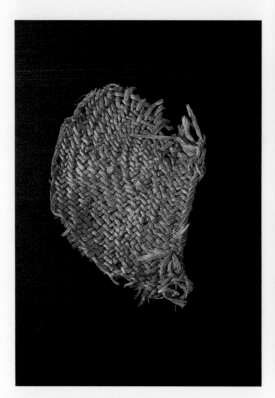

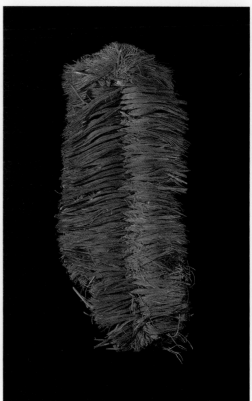

172   *Catalog no.:* 2831
Site: Twin Cave House, Arizona
Collector and date: Byron Cummings, University of
    Utah Expedition, 1913
Cultural period: Pueblo II-Pueblo III
Construction technique: Plaited
Dimensions: Length 17.0 cm, width 12.0 cm, depth
    0.76 cm
Active elements: Leaf element, unspun, cortex intact
Average width: 0.31 cm
Passive elements: N/A
Ties, loops, attachments: Edge: Leaf remnant
Shape: Left foot shaping, tapered toe with jog, heel
    missing
Start: Appears active elements folded with addition
    of a folded element for toe jog
Body: 2/2 twill plaiting with a 2/3/2 shift on selvages.
    Three long stitches appear to be single stitches
    with ends left frayed on sole. Exhausted ends
    frayed on sole
Other: Structural padding on heel

Catalog no.: 2832
Site: Twin Cave House, Arizona
Collector and date: Byron Cummings, University of
    Utah Expedition, 1913
Cultural period: Unknown
Construction technique: Plain weave
Dimensions: Length 23.0 cm, width 10.5 cm, depth
    1.31 cm
Active elements: Leaf element unspun, cortex intact
Average width: 0.35 cm
Passive elements: Leaf element unspun, cortex intact
Number of passive units: 2
Number in unit: 3(?)
Average width: 0.71 cm
Ties, loops, attachments: A loose knot rests on top
    of sandal.
Shape: Rounded toe and heel
Start: Warps are tied together at toe in one knot.
Body: Over-under plain weave beginning with
    narrow ends of leaf element on top and ending
    with shredded wide ends on sole for padding.
    Ends extend beyond body of sandal, increasing
    width.
Finish: At heel warp ends tied in one knot
Other: Structural padding on sole

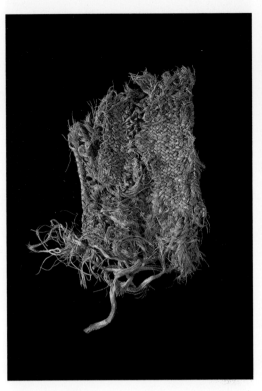

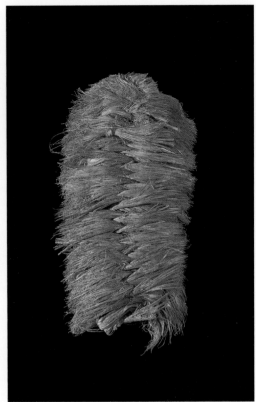

Catalog no.: 2833
Site: Twin Cave House, Arizona
Collector and date: Byron Cummings, University of
Utah Expedition, 1913
Cultural period: Pueblo II-Pueblo III
Construction technique: Plaited
Dimensions: Length 15.5 cm, width 9.75 cm, depth
1.02 cm
Active elements: Leaf element, unspun, cortex intact
Average width: Top: 0.17 cm Bottom: 0.29 cm
Passive elements: N/A
Ties, loops, attachments: Edge: Remnants of loops,
one knot
Shape: Unknown, toe and heel missing, fragmentary
Start and Finish: Missing
Body: 2/2 twill plaiting on both layers of joined
sandals
Other: Two sandals bound together by six rows of
stitching running from toe to heel

Catalog no.: 2834
Site: Twin Cave House, Arizona
Collector and date: Byron Cummings, University of
Utah Expedition, 1913
Cultural period: Unknown
Construction technique: Plain weave
Dimensions: Length 21.5 cm, width 11.0 cm, depth
1.50 cm
Active elements: Leaf element unspun, cortex intact
Average width: 0.43 cm
Passive elements: Leaf element unspun, cortex intact
Number of passive units: 2
Number in unit: 3(?)
Average width: 0.79 cm
Ties, loops, attachments: None apparent
Shape: Rounded toe and heel incomplete
Start: Warps are tied together at toe in one knot.
Body: Over-under plain weave beginning with
narrow ends of leaf element on top and ending
with shredded wide ends on sole for padding.
Wefts encircle warps both tightly and loosely,
which extends the width of sandal beyond the
warp edge.
Finish: Missing
Other: Structural padding on sole

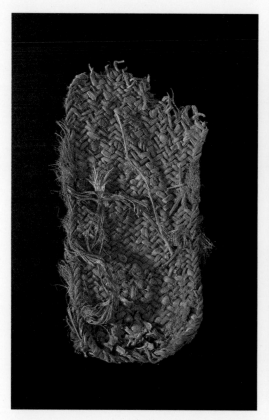
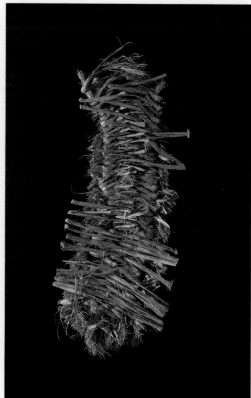

Catalog no.: 2835

Site: Twin Cave House, Arizona

Collector and date: Byron Cummings, University of
Utah Expedition, 1913

Cultural period: Pueblo II-Pueblo III

Construction technique: Plaited

Dimensions: Length 20.2 cm, width 9.8 cm, depth
1.15 cm

Active elements: Leaf element, unspun, cortex intact

Average width: 0.60 cm

Passive elements: N/A

Ties, loops, attachments: Edge: Two edge loops
remain of shredded leaf fiber on left side. Knots
on both sides of 2 ply, s-Z twist cordage. Heel:
Two remnant knots.

Shape: Left foot shaping, rounded heel, toe missing

Start: Missing

Body: 2/2 twill plaiting with a 2/3/2 shift at selvages
Exhausted ends left frayed on sole

Finish: At heel ends protrude on surface of sandal.

Other: Additional stitches appear added for
structure with ends left frayed on sole. Structual
padding on sole.

Catalog no.: 2836

Site: Twin Cave House, Arizona

Collector and date: Byron Cummings, University of
Utah Expedition, 1913

Cultural period: Unknown

Construction technique: Plain weave

Dimensions: Length 25.0 cm, width 6.5 cm, depth
1.9 cm

Active elements: Leaf element unspun, cortex intact

Average width: 0.39 cm

Passive elements: Leaf element unspun, cortex intact

Number of passive units: 2

Number in unit: 1(?)

Average width: 0.32 cm

Ties, loops, attachments: None apparent

Shape: Rounded finished end

Start or Finish: Warps are tied in one knot at toe.

Body: Over-under plain weave beginning with
narrow ends of leaf element on top and ending
with shredded wide ends on sole for padding.
Ends extend beyond body of sandal, increasing
width.

Other: Structural padding on sole

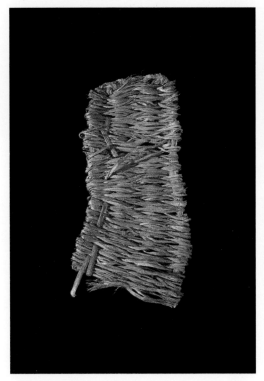
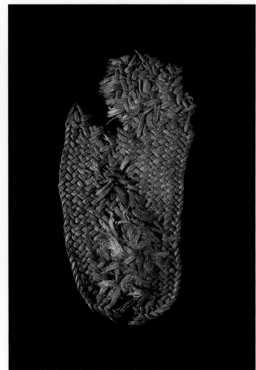

Catalog no.: 2837
Site: Twin Cave House, Arizona
Collector and date: Byron Cummings, University of
  Utah Expedition, 1909
Cultural period: Unknown
Construction technique: Plain weave
Dimensions: Length 17.45 cm, width 8.87 cm, depth
  0.85 cm
Active elements: Leaf element unspun, cortex intact
Average width: 0.30 cm
Passive elements: Leaf element unspun, cortex intact
Number of passive units: 4
Number in unit: 2
Average width: 0.58 cm
Ties, loops, attachments: None apparent
Shape: Squared heel, toe missing
Start: Missing
Body: Over-under plain weave for length of sandal
  beginning with narrow end of leaf element and
  ending with shredded wide ends on sole for
  padding
Other: Structural padding on sole

Catalog no.: 2838
Site: Twin Cave House, Arizona
Collector and date: Byron Cummings, University of
  Utah Expedition, 1913
Cultural period: Pueblo II-Pueblo III
Construction technique: Plaited
Dimensions: Length 20.8 cm, width 10.3 cm, depth
  0.80 cm
Active elements: Leaf element, unspun, cortex intact
Average width: 0.42 cm
Passive elements: N/A
Ties, loops, attachments: None apparent
Shape: Left foot shaping, round heel, toe missing
Start: Missing
Body: 2/2 twill plaiting for length of sandal
Finish: Undeterminable due to disarticulation
Other: Heavy mending with leaf elements in central
  area from heel to toe.

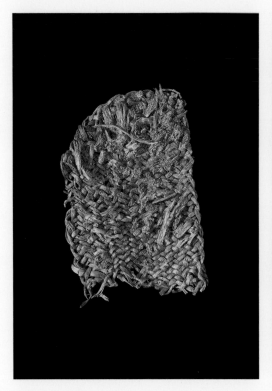
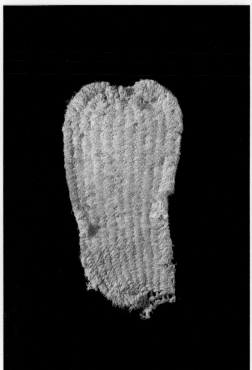

176 *Catalog no.:* 2839
Site: Twin Cave House, Arizona
Collector and date: Byron Cummings, University of
Utah Expedition, 1913
Cultural period: Pueblo II-Pueblo III
Construction technique: Plaited
Dimensions: Length 16.6 cm, width 11.0 cm, depth
0.90 cm
Active elements: Leaf element, unspun, cortex intact
Average width: 0.33 cm
Passive elements: N/A
Ties, loops, attachments: None apparent
Shape: Right foot shaping, tapered toe with jog,
heel missing
Start: Active elements folded at toe with addition
of folded element at toe jog
Body: 2/2 twill plaiting with irregular shifts at toe
for shaping. 2/1/2 shifts at selvage. Exhausted
ends frayed on sole
Finish: Missing
Other: Structural padding on sole

Catalog no.: 2840
Site: Twin Cave House, Arizona
Collector and date: Byron Cummings, University of
Utah Expedition, 1913
Cultural period: Unknown
Construction technique: Plain weave and twined
Dimensions: Length 18.1 cm, width 9.7 cm, depth
0.8 cm
Active elements: Cordage, element 2 ply, z-S twist
Average width: 0.25 cm
Passive elements: Cordage, element 2 ply, z-S twist
Number of passive units: 10(?)
Number in unit: 1
Average width: 0.23 cm
Ties, loops, attachments: Remnants of cordage worn
flush with sandal appear on both sides of toe,
instep, and edge.
Shape: Left foot shaping, heart shaped toe, heel
missing
Start: It appears 5(?) elements were folded at toe
to form 10(?) warps. The arrangement appears
to be that edge warps cross over each other at
the center; another element folds at center
crossing the first two warps; and two warps are
folded (one on each side) inside the outer edge
warp.
Body: 2/2 alternate pair twining for forward section
of sandal. Remaining portion over-under plain
weave
Finish: Missing

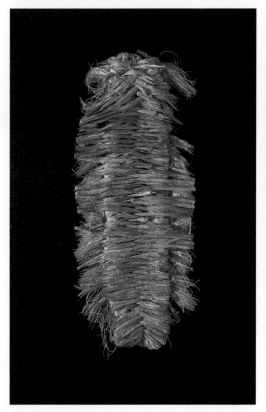

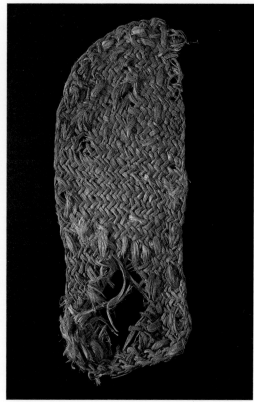

Catalog no.: 2842
Site: Twin Cave House, Arizona
Collector and date: Byron Cummings, University of
    Utah Expedition, 1913
Cultural period: Unknown
Construction technique: Plain weave
Dimensions: Length 22.0 cm, width 9.0 cm, depth
    1.0 cm
Active elements: Leaf element unspun, cortex intact
Average width: 0.43 cm
Passive elements: Leaf element unspun, cortex intact
Number of passive units: 2
Number in unit: 3
Average width: 0.63 cm
Ties, loops, attachments: Toe: One leaf element
    crosses wefts and pierces sole.
Shape: Rounded toe and heel
Start: Warps are tied together at toe in two knots.
Body: Over-under plain weave beginning with
    narrow ends of leaf element on top and ending
    with shredded wide ends on sole for padding.
    Ends extend beyond body of sandal, increasing
    width.
Finish: At heel warps are tied in two knots.
Other: Structural padding on sole

Catalog no.: 3141
Site: Twin Cave House, Arizona
Collector and date: Byron Cummings, University of
    Utah Expedition, 1913
Cultural period: Pueblo II-Pueblo III
Construction technique: Plaited
Dimensions: Length 31.2 cm, width 11.2 cm, depth
    0.57 cm
Active elements: Leaf element, unspun, cortex intact
Average width: 0.29 cm
Passive elements: N/A
Ties, loops, attachments: None apparent
Shape: Left foot shaping, tapered toe, squared heel
Start: Active elements folded at toe
Body: 2/2 twill plaiting for length of sandal with
    shifts of 2/1/2 in middle of sandal
Finish: At heel ends appear looped around adjacent
    elements.
Other: Stitching on sandal appears to be structural.

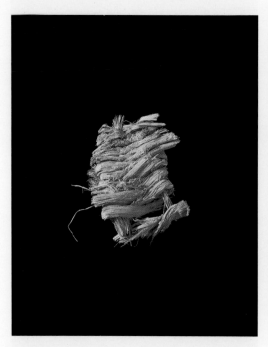
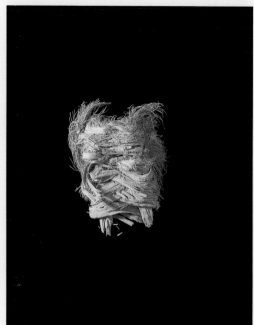

178   *Catalog no.:* 42SΛ373 (FS9.20 A) 24048
Site: Wasp House, Utah
Collector and date: UCRBASP, 1960
Cultural period: Pueblo II-Pueblo III
Construction technique: Plain weave
Dimensions: Length 9.9 cm, width 5.6 cm, depth 1.3 cm
Active elements: Leaf element, unspun, cortex intact
Average width: 0.35 cm
Passive elements: Leaf element unspun, cortex intact
Number of passive units: 2
Number in unit: 1
Average width: 1.0 cm
Ties, loops, attachments: None apparent
Shape: Fragmentary
Start or Finish: Warps are tied together in one knot at toe. Only one end present
Body: Over-under plain weave beginning with narrow ends of leaf element on top and ending with shredded wide ends on sole for padding. Ends extend beyond body of sandal.
Other: Structural padding on sole

Catalog no.: 42SA373 (FS9.20 B) 24048
Site: Wasp House, Utah
Collector and date: UCRBASP, 1960
Cultural period: Pueblo II-Pueblo III
Construction technique: Plain weave
Dimensions: Length 10.0 cm, width 7.0 cm, depth 1.5 cm
Active elements: Leaf element, unspun, cortex intact
Average width: 0.6 cm
Passive elements: Leaf element unspun, cortex intact
Number of passive units: 2
Number in unit: 1
Average width: 0.93 cm
Ties, loops, attachments: None apparent
Shape: Fragmentary
Start or Finish: Warps are tied together in one knot at toe. Only one end present
Body: Over-under plain weave beginning with narrow ends of leaf element on top and ending with shredded wide ends on sole for padding. Ends extend beyond body of sandal.
Other: Structural padding on sole

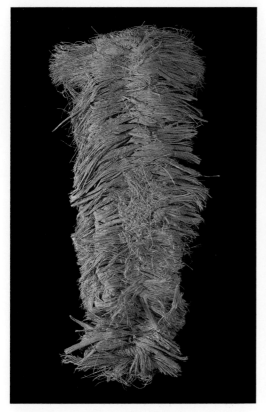
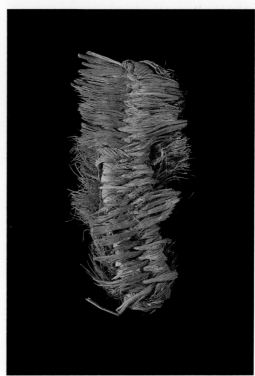

Catalog no.: 42SA633 (FS12.2) 24131
Site: Widow's Ledge, Utah
Collector and date: UCRBASP, 1962
Cultural period: Pueblo II-Pueblo III
Construction technique: Plain weave
Dimensions: Length 27.0 cm, width 12.5 cm, depth 1.2 cm
Active elements: Leaf element unspun, cortex intact
Average width: 0.60 cm
Passive elements: Leaf element unspun, cortex intact
Number of passive units: 2
Number in unit: 1(?)
Average width: 0.80 cm
Ties, loops, attachments: Unknown
Shape: Squared toe and heel
Start: Two warps tied together at toe in one knot
Body: Over-under plain weave beginning with narrow ends of leaf element on top and ending with shredded wide ends on sole for padding. Ends extend beyond body of sandal.
Finish: At heel warps are tied in one knot.
Other: Structural padding on sole

Catalog no.: 42SA633 (FS12.8) 24131
Site: Widow's Ledge, Utah
Collector and date: UCRBASP, 1962
Cultural period: Pueblo II-Pueblo III
Construction technique: Plain weave
Dimensions: Length 19.3 cm, width 8.50 cm, depth 1.3 cm
Active elements: Leaf element unspun, cortex intact
Average width: 0.56 cm
Passive elements: Leaf element unspun, cortex intact
Number of passive units: 2
Number in unit: 2-3
Average width: 0.84 cm
Ties, loops, attachments: None apparent
Shape: Straight toe, heel missing
Start: Warps are tied together at toe in three knots.
Body: Over-under plain weave for length of sandal with ends extending beyond width of sandal
Finish: Missing
Other: Structural padding on sole

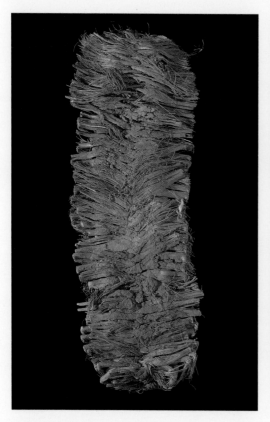
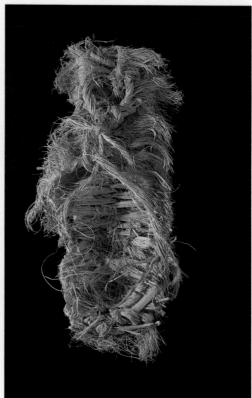

180 *Catalog no.:* 42SA633 (FS28.31) 24131
Site: Widow's Ledge, Utah
Collector and date: UCRBASP, 1962
Cultural period: Pueblo II-Pueblo III
Construction technique: Plain weave
Dimensions: Length 27.7 cm, width 11.0 cm, depth 0.85 cm
Active elements: Leaf element unspun, cortex intact
Average width: 0.41 cm
Passive elements: Leaf element unspun, cortex intact
Number of passive units: 2
Number in unit: 1(?)
Average width: 0.93 cm
Ties, loops, attachments: None apparent
Shape: Squared toe and heel
Start: Two leaf elements tied together at toe in one knot
Body: Over-under plain weave beginning with narrow ends of leaf element on top and ending with shredded wide ends on sole for padding. Welts and ends extend beyond warp edge of sandal.
Finish: At heel warps are tied in three knots.
Other: Structural padding on sole

Catalog no.: 42SA633 (FS30.7) 24131
Site: Widow's Ledge, Utah
Collector and date: UCRBASP, 1962
Cultural period: Pueblo II-Pueblo III
Construction technique: Plain weave
Dimensions: Length 24.0 cm, width 8.5 cm, depth 1.32 cm
Active elements: Leaf element unspun, cortex intact
Average width: 0.50 cm
Passive elements: Leaf element unspun, cortex intact
Number of passive units: 2
Number in unit: 1(?)
Average width: 0.76 cm
Ties, loops, attachments: None apparent
Shape: Rounded toe and heel
Start: Two warps tied together at toe in one knot
Body: Over-under plain weave beginning with narrow ends of leaf element on top and ending with shredded wide ends on sole for padding. Ends extend beyond body of sandal.
Finish: Warps tied together in two knots at heel
Other: Structural padding on sole

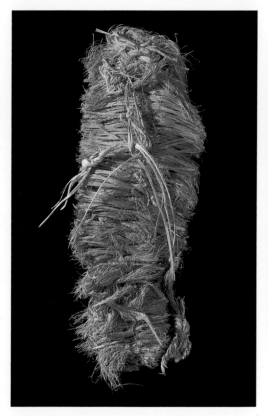

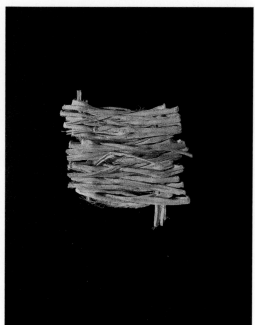

Catalog no.: 42SA633 (FS30.8) 24131
Site: Widow's Ledge, Utah
Collector and date: UCRBASP, 1962
Cultural period: Pueblo II-Pueblo III
Construction technique: Plain weave
Dimensions: Length 27.0 cm, width 10 cm, depth 1.4 cm
Active elements: Leaf element unspun, cortex intact
Average width: 0.55 cm
Passive elements: Leaf element unspun, cortex intact
Number of passive units: 2
Number in unit: 1
Average width: 0.87 cm
Ties, loops, attachments: Toe: Loop, S twist, passes under sole and ties on top. Heel: Remnant of loop, S twist. Heel loop knotted to loop that extends to toe
Shape: Rounded toe and heel
Start: Warps are tied together at toe in one knot.
Body: Over-under plain weave beginning with narrow ends of leaf element on top and ending with shredded wide ends on sole for padding. Wefts encircle warps both tightly and loosely which extends the width of sandal beyond the warp edge. Ends extend beyond body of sandal.
Finish: At heel warps are knotted in one knot.
Other: Structural padding on sole

Catalog no.: 42SA633 (FS34.8) 24131   181
Site: Widow's Ledge, Utah
Collector and date: UCRBASP, 1962
Cultural period: Pueblo II-Pueblo III
Construction technique: Plain weave
Dimensions: Length 7.50 cm, width 9.20 cm, depth 0.40 cm
Active elements: Leaf element unspun, cortex intact
Average width: 0.32 cm
Passive elements: Leaf element unspun, cortex intact
Number of passive units: 2
Number in unit: 1(?)
Average width: 0.61 cm
Ties, loops, attachments: None apparent
Shape: Fragmentary
Start: Missing
Body: Over-under plain weave beginning with narrow ends of leaf element on top and ending with shredded wide ends on sole for padding
Finish: Missing
Other: Structural padding on sole

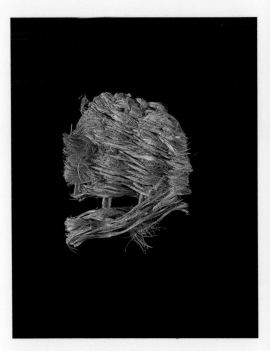

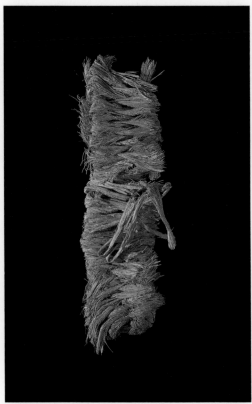

182   *Catalog no.:* 42SA633 (FS35.23)
Site: Widow's Ledge, Utah
Collector and date: UCRBASP, 1962
Cultural period: Pueblo II-Pueblo III
Construction technique: Plain weave
Dimensions: Length 8.51 cm, width 9.63 cm, depth
1.38 cm
Active elements: Leaf element unspun, cortex intact
Average width: 0.43 cm
Passive elements: Leaf element unspun, cortex intact
Number of passive units: 4
Number in unit: 2 (?)
Average width: 0.61 cm
Ties, loops, attachments: None apparent
Shape: Fragmentary
Start or Finish: Six parallel elements are knotted into
3 knots. The two inside warps are woven
double.
Body: Over-under plain weave beginning with
narrow ends of leaf element on top and ending
with shredded wide ends on sole for padding
Other: Structural padding on sole

Catalog no.: 42SA633 (FS43.18A) 24131
Site: Widow's Ledge, Utah
Collector and date: UCRBASP, 1962
Cultural period: Pueblo II-Pueblo III
Construction technique: Plain weave
Dimensions: Length 22.0 cm, width 6.0 cm, depth
1.35 cm
Active elements: Leaf element unspun, cortex intact
Average width: 0.46 cm
Passive elements: Leaf element unspun, cortex intact
Number of passive units: 2
Number in unit: 1
Average width: 0.82 cm
Ties, loops, attachments: None apparent
Shape: Fragmentary
Start or Finish: Two warps are tied together in one
knot at toe.
Body: Over-under plain weave beginning with
narrow ends of leaf element on top and ending
with shredded wide ends on sole for padding
Other: Structural padding on sole

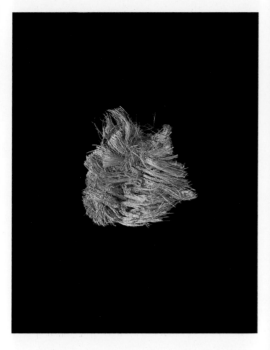

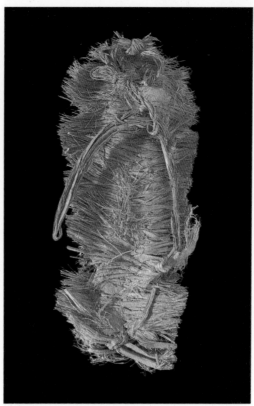

Catalog no.: 42SA633 (FS43.18B) 24131
Site: Widow's Ledge, Utah
Collector and date: UCRBASP, 1962
Cultural period: Pueblo II-Pueblo III
Construction technique: Plain weave
Dimensions: Length 9.0 cm, width 8.5 cm, depth 1.15 cm
Active elements: Leaf element unspun, cortex intact
Average width: 0.36 cm
Passive elements: Leaf element unspun, cortex intact
Number of passive units: 2
Number in unit: 1
Average width: 0.86 cm
Ties, loops, attachments: None apparent
Shape: Fragmentary
Start or Finish: Two warps are tied in one knot at toe.
Body: Over-under plain weave beginning with narrow leaf element on top and ending with shredded wide ends on sole for padding
Other: Structural padding on sole

Catalog no.: 42SA633 (FS48.3) 24131
Site: Widow's Ledge, Utah
Collector and date: UCRBASP, 1962
Cultural period: Pueblo II-Pueblo III
Construction technique: Plain weave
Dimensions: Length 26.0 cm, width 12.0 cm, depth 1.5 cm
Active elements: Leaf element unspun, cortex intact
Average width: 0.54 cm
Passive elements: Leaf element unspun, cortex intact
Number of passive units: 2
Number in unit: 3(?)
Average width: 0.82 cm
Ties, loops, attachments: Toe and Edge: Cordage, loop 2 ply, s-Z twist, loops through a leaf tie at toe and longer tie that extends on both sides to ankle area where it is still attached to edge on left side
Shape: Rounded toe and squared heel
Start: Three warps are tied in one knot at toe.
Body: Over-under plain weave beginning with narrow ends of leaf element on top and ending with shredded wide ends on sole for padding. Ends extend beyond body of sandal.
Finish: At heel three separate knots draw warps back together.
Other: Structural padding on sole

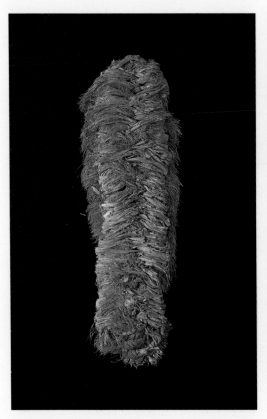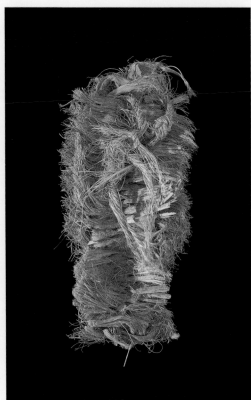

184 *Catalog no.:* 42SA633 (FS55.7) 24131
Site: Widow's Ledge, Utah
Collector and date: UCRBASP, 1962
Cultural period: Pueblo II-Pueblo III
Construction technique: Plain weave
Dimensions: Length 22.0 cm, width 10.0, depth 1.3 cm
Active elements: Leaf element unspun, cortex intact
Average width: 0.50 cm
Passive elements: Leaf element unspun, cortex intact
Number of passive units: 2
Number in unit: 2
Average width: 0.93 cm
Ties, loops, attachments: Toe: Leaf element twisted Z looped through wefts at toe and knotted with a square knot. Edges: Loop of slightly S twisted leaf element at instep encircles toe loop and loop that extends to both edges of sandal near heel.
Shape: Slightly squared toe and heel
Start: Two warps are tied in one knot at toe.
Body: Over-under plain weave beginning with narrow ends of leaf element on top and ending with shredded wide ends on sole for padding
Finish: At heel two separate knots draw warps back together.
Other: Structural padding on sole

Catalog no.: 42SA633 (FS55.8) 24131
Site: Widow's Ledge, Utah
Collector and date: UCRBASP, 1962
Cultural period: Pueblo II-Pueblo III
Construction technique: Plain weave
Dimensions: Length 23.0 cm, width 11.0 cm, depth 1.10 cm
Active elements: Leaf element unspun, cortex intact
Average width: 0.58 cm
Passive elements: Leaf element unspun, cortex intact
Number of passive units: 2
Number in unit: 1(?)
Average width: 0.78 cm
Ties, loops, attachments: Toe: Loop is formed with two separate elements each attached to a warp, then shredded and twisted Z and tied in a square knot. Additional loops are looped through one another and tied. Edge: S twist loops at instep attach to toe loop.
Shape: Rounded toe
Start: Two warps tied together at toe in one knot
Body: Over-under plain weave beginning with narrow ends of leaf element on top and ending with shredded wide ends on sole for padding. Ends extend beyond body of sandal.
Finish: At heel warps are tied in two knots.
Other: Structural padding on sole

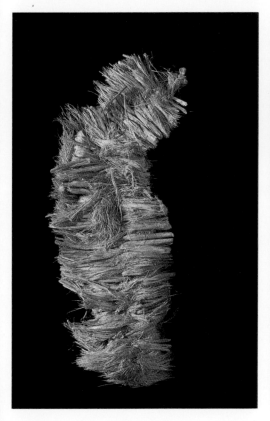
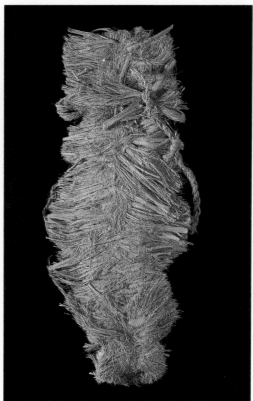

Catalog no.: 42SA633 (FS59.20) 24131
Site: Widow's Ledge, Utah
Collector and date: UCRBASP, 1962
Cultural period: Pueblo II-Pueblo III
Construction technique: Plain weave
Dimensions: Length 26.0 cm, width 9.5 cm, depth 2.2 cm
Active elements: Leaf element unspun, cortex intact
Average width: 0.5 cm
Passive elements: Leaf element unspun, cortex intact
Number of passive units: 2
Number in unit: 1
Average width: 0.72 cm
Ties, loops, attachments: None apparent
Shape: Rounded toe and heel
Start: Warps are tied together at toe in one large knot.
Body: Over-under plain weave beginning with narrow ends of leaf element on top and ending with shredded wide ends on sole for padding. Wefts encircle warps both tightly and loosely which extends the width of sandal beyond the warp edge. Ends also extend beyond body of sandal.
Finish: Heel end finished with 2 knots, in sequence, of warp elements
Other: Structural padding on sole

Catalog no.: 42SA633 (FS59.21) 24131
Site: Widow's Ledge, Utah
Collector and date: UCRBASP, 1962
Cultural period: Pueblo II-Pueblo III
Construction technique: Plain weave
Dimensions: Length 27.0 cm, width 11.0 cm, depth 1.10 cm
Active elements: Leaf element unspun, cortex intact
Average width: 0.30 cm
Passive elements: Leaf element unspun, cortex intact
Number of passive units: 2
Number in unit: 1(?)
Average width: 0.5 cm
Ties, loops, attachments: Toe: Leaf element tie. Heel: S twist leaf element tie. Edge: At one edge 2 cords loop and tie, 2 ply s-Z twist. Other edge cord remnants, 2 ply s-Z twist
Shape: Rounded toe and squared heel
Start: Two warps tied together at toe in one knot
Body: Over-under plain weave beginning with narrow ends of leaf element on top and ending with shredded wide ends on sole for padding. Ends extend beyond body of sandal.
Finish: Warp ends tied in one knot
Other: Structural padding on sole

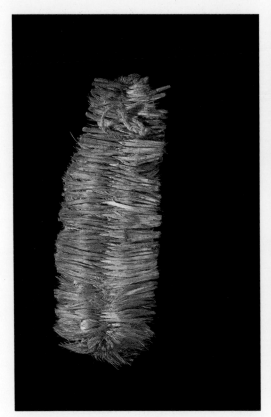
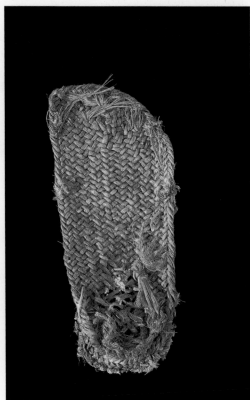

186 *Catalog no.:* AR326 85.1
Site: Unknown
Collector and date: Probably Byron Cummings
collection
Cultural period: Unknown
Construction technique: Plain weave
Dimensions: Length 22.0 cm, width 8.5 cm, depth
1.2 cm
Active elements: Leaf element unspun, cortex intact
Average width: 0.29 cm
Passive elements: Leaf element unspun, cortex intact
Number of passive units: 2
Number in unit: 1
Average width: 0.45 cm
Ties, loops, attachments: Heel: Cordage, 2 ply, s-Z
twist
Shape: Rounded toe and heel
Start: Warps tied together at toe in one knot
Body: Over-under plain weave beginning with
narrow ends of leaf element on top and ending
with shredded wide ends on sole for padding.
Wefts encircle warps both tightly and loosely
which extends the width of sandal beyond the
warp edge.
Finish: At heel warps are tied in one knot.
Other: Structural padding on sole

Catalog no.: AR334 85.1
Site: Unknown
Collector and date: Probably Byron Cummings
collection
Cultural period: Unknown
Construction technique: Plaited
Dimensions: Length 24.0 cm, width 10.5 cm, depth
0.87 cm
Active elements: Leaf element unspun, cortex intact
Average width: 0.43 cm
Passive elements: N/A
Ties, loops, attachments: Toe: Leaf fragments, one tie
still intact. Heel: Cordage tripled back and forth
at heel. First row is single ply tucked tightly
under cupped heel. Next two cords are 2 ply
s-Z twist that doubles around heel tie which is
knotted to an edge tie.
Shape: Right foot shaping, tapered toe and rounded
heel
Start: Active elements folded at toe. Folded
elements added as tapering widens sandal
Body: 2/2 twill plaiting for length of sandal with
shifts at toe, heel and center of 2/1/2 and 2/3/
1/2 for shaping. Edges are pulled in with a 2/3/2
shift. Exhausted ends left frayed on sole.
Finish: At heel plaiting is pulled tight to create a
thick rolled selvage. Active elements are knotted
with ends protruding on back of heel and sole.
Other: Structural padding on sole.

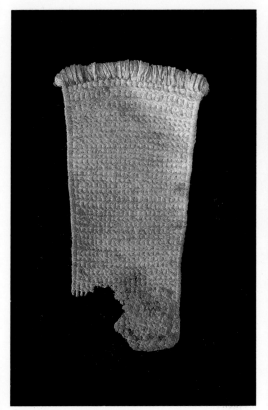 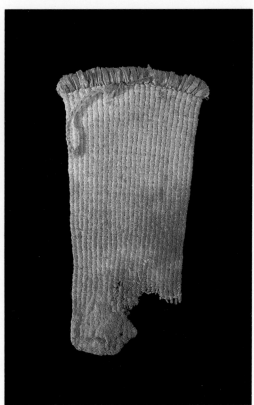

Catalog no.: AR327 85.1
Site: Unknown
Collector and date: Probably Byron Cummings
   Collection
Cultural period: Basketmaker II(?)
Construction technique: Composite
Dimensions: Length 23.0 cm, width 13.0 cm, depth
   0.45 cm
Active elements: Cordage, 2 ply, z-S twist
Average width: 0.22 cm
Passive elements: Cordage, 3 ply, z-S twist
Number of passive units: 26
Number in unit: 1
Average width: 0.33 cm
Ties, loops, attachments: Toe: Cordage, 2 ply, s-Z twist,
   remnant on right side. Hide wrapping at toe.
Shape: Squared toe and heel
Start: At toe warps are aligned parallel with ends
   left exposed or folded over a rigid element
   secured from two points. It appears there is one
   row of twining. Additional leaf material is
   wrapped over twining and between warps with a
   final wrapping of hide to bind elements.
Body: Beginning at toe and repeating 3 times, there
   are four rows of plain weave and two soumac or
   one chained row. Remainder of sandal to heel
   repeats pattern of several rows of plain weave
   and one row of soumac either to the right or
   left, which varies the stitch slant. At heel there
   appear to be supplemental wefts which wrap
   around warp and weft to create a raised pattern.
Finish: At heel warps appear folded to sole side,
   then twined with ends tucked in.
Other: Charring at heel

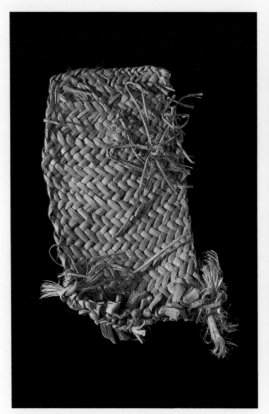 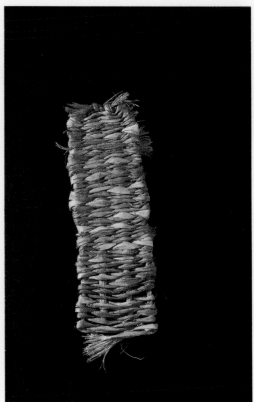

188   *Catalog no.:* AR533 86.1

Site: Unknown

Collector and date: Probably Byron Cummings
Collection

Cultural period: Unknown

Construction technique: Plaited

Dimensions: Length 20.5 cm, width 10.30 cm, depth
0.93 cm

Active elements: Leaf element unspun, cortex intact

Average width: 0.50 cm

Passive elements: N/A

Ties, loops, attachments: Toe: Leaf element tie
inserted into sandal at both edges

Heel: Leaf element remnant ties

Edge: Knotted leaf elements loop through other
elements on left side.

Shape: Right foot shaping, rounded toe and heel

Start: Active elements doubled and aligned parallel.
Twining near top of elements to anchor with
short ends above twining. Elements are then
folded, which covers one side of twining.

Body: 2/2 twill plaiting on doubled ends for a
distance of 2.2 cm at which point doubled
elements are dropped and plaiting is with single
elements. Shifts of 2/1/2 for shaping

Finish: A transverse element makes a loop at heel.
Active elements alternately wrap on upper part
of loop and lower part of loop.

Catalog no.: AR535 86.1

Site: Unknown

Collector and date: Probably Byron Cummings
Collection

Cultural period: Unknown

Construction technique: Plain weave

Dimensions: Length 18.0 cm, width 6.0 cm, depth
1.0 cm

Active elements: Leaf element, unspun, cortex intact

Average width: 0.49 cm

Passive elements: Leaf element unspun, cortex intact

Number of passive units: 4

Number in unit: 1

Average width: 0.45 cm

Ties, loops, attachments: None apparent

Shape: Rounded finished end

Start or Finish: Warps are knotted in two groups
then middle two warps are knotted in a third
group.

Body: Over-under plain weave for length of sandal.
Wide ends left shredded on sole for padding

Other: Structural padding on sole

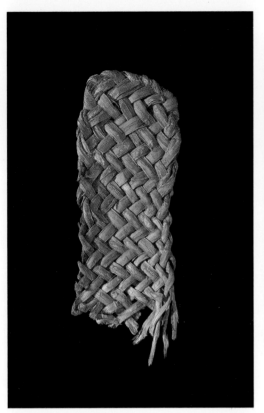

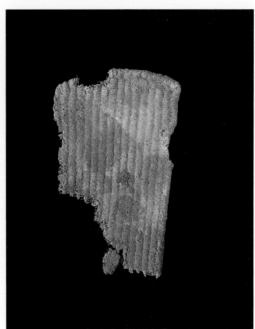

Catalog no.: AR536 86.1
Site: Unknown
Collector and date: Probably Byron Cummings
  collection
Cultural period: Unknown
Construction technique: Plaited
Dimensions: Length 19.5 cm, width 8.3 cm, depth
  0.90 cm
Active elements: Leaf element unspun, cortex intact
Average width: 0.72 cm
Passive elements: N/A
Ties, loops, attachments: None apparent
Shape: Rounded at toe, fragmentary
Start: Doubled active elements are folded at toe.
Body: 2/2 twill weaving on doubled elements for
  approximately one-third of sandal. Doubled
  elements end and remainder of sandal is woven
  with single elements.
Finish: Missing

Catalog no.: AR730 86.1
Site: Unknown
Collector and date: Probably Byron Cummings
  collection
Cultural period: Basketmaker II (?)
Construction technique: Composite
Dimensions: Length 16.0 cm, width 10.5 cm, depth
  0.65 cm
Active elements: Cordage, 2 ply, z-S twist
Average width: 0.15 cm
Passive elements: Cordage, 2 ply, z-S twist
Number of passive units: 16
Number in unit: 2
Average width: 0.28 cm
Ties, loops, attachments: None apparent
Shape: Squared toe, fragmentary
Start: Elements appear doubled at toe with a row
  of twining visible on upper surface only. It is
  possible warps were aligned parallel, twined,
  then folded over a rigid element suspended from
  two points.
Body: 1/1 plain weave over doubled warps for
  length of sandal in combination with warp
  wrapping to give raised ribs on sole
Finish: Missing

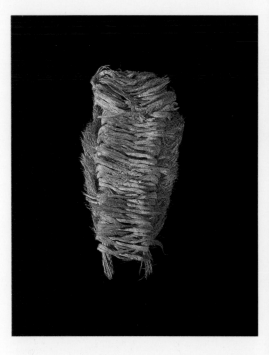

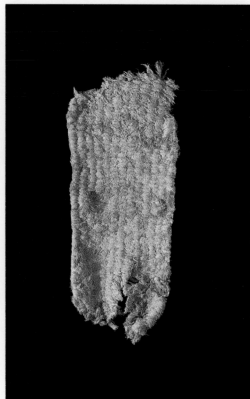

190 *Catalog no.:* AR769 86.1
Site: Unknown
Collector and date: Probably Byron Cummings
   collection
Cultural period: Unknown
Construction technique: Plain weave
Dimensions: Length 15.88 cm, width 7.73 cm, depth
   1.15 cm
Active elements: Leaf element unspun, cortex intact
Average width: 0.43 cm
Passive elements: Leaf element unspun, cortex intact
Number of passive units: 2
Number in unit: 2
Average width: 0.52 cm
Ties, loops, attachments: None apparent
Shape: Rounded finished end
Start or Finish: Warps are tied together in two
   knots at toe.
Body: Over-under plain weave beginning with
   narrow ends of leaf element on top and ending
   with shredded wide ends on sole for padding
Other: Structural padding on sole

Catalog no.: AR777 86.1
Site: Unknown
Collector and date: Probably Byron Cummings
   collection
Cultural period: Unknown
Construction technique: Plain weave
Dimensions: Length 22.0 cm, width 9.0 cm, depth
   0.68 cm
Active elements: Cordage, 2 ply, z-S twist
Average width: 0.35 cm
Passive elements: Cordage, 2 ply, z-S twist
Number of passive units: 13
Number in unit: 1
Average width: 0.30 cm
Ties, loops, attachments: Heel: Two cordage knots 2
   ply, z-S twist(?) near one edge. Edge: Stubs
   protrude on both edges.
Shape: Unknown, possible puckered heel
Start: Missing
Body: Over-under plain weave for length of sandal
Finish: Possible puckered heel. One warp turns back
   into upper surface of sandal.

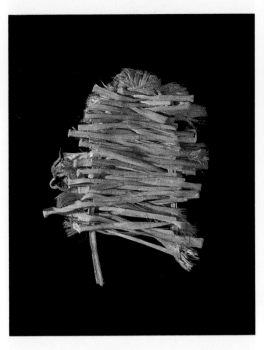

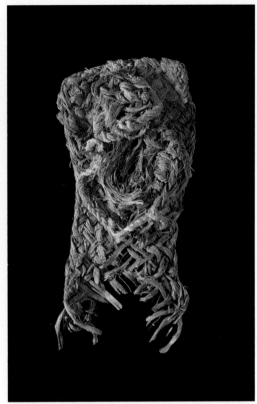

Catalog no.: AR778 86.1
Site: Unknown
Collector and date: Probably Byron Cummings
   collection
Cultural period: Unknown
Construction technique: Plain weave
Dimensions: Length 17.0 cm, width 11.0 cm, depth
   1.8 cm
Active elements: Leaf element unspun, cortex intact
Average width: 0.46 cm
Passive elements: Leaf element unspun, cortex intact
Number of passive units: 2
Number in unit: 2
Average width: 0.60 cm
Ties, loops, attachments: None apparent
Shape: Rounded finished end
Start or Finish: Warps are tied together in two
   knots at toe and wrapped.
Body: Over-under plain weave beginning with
   narrow ends of leaf element on top and ending
   with shredded wide ends on sole for padding.
   Wefts encircle warps both tightly and loosely,
   which along with extended frayed ends increases
   width of sandal.
Other: Structural padding on sole

Catalog no.: AR780 86.1
Site: Unknown
Collector and date: Probably Byron Cummings
   collection
Cultural period: Unknown
Construction technique: Plaited
Dimensions: Length 22.50 cm, width 11.0 cm, depth
   1.25 cm
Active elements: Leaf element unspun, cortex intact
Average width: 0.48 cm
Passive elements: N/A
Ties, loops, attachments: Toe: Cordage 2 ply, s-Z
   twist is looped through weaving on both sides
   and twisted back on itself to form a 4 ply.
Shape: Squared toe, heel missing
Start: Active elements folded at toe. Horizontal
   row of twining 2.0 cm from toe with 2 ply, s-Z
   twist cordage knotted at both edges
Body: 2/2 twill plaiting for length of sandal. What
   appear to be stitches are not connected.
   Elements are stitched on surface with both ends
   knotted on sole to active elements which create
   large bumps.
Finish: Heel missing
Other: A heel portion of a separate sandal complete
   with heel loop has been inserted under toe loop.
   It is possible this is the missing heel section of
   this sandal.

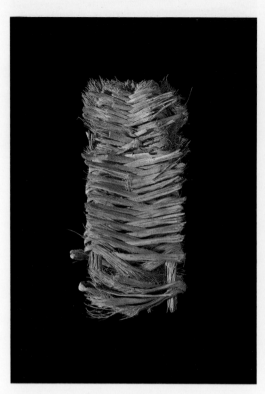

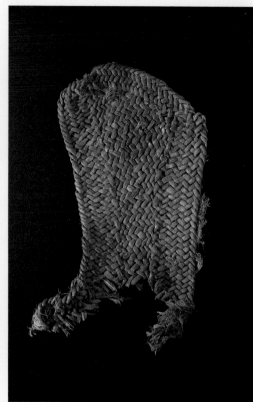

Catalog no.: AR829 86.1
Site: Unknown
Collector and date: Probably Byron Cummings
  collection
Cultural period: Unknown
Construction technique: Plaited
Dimensions: Length 21.0 cm, width 11.4 cm, depth
  0.50 cm
Active elements: Leaf element, unspun, cortex intact
Average width: 0.54 cm
Passive elements: N/A
Ties, loops, attachments: None. Possible awl hole on
  left side near heel for attachment
Shape: Right foot shaping. Tapered toe with little
  toe jog. Heel missing
Start: Elements appear folded at toe, with elements
  added as necessary for tapering and toe jog.
Body: 2/2 twill plaiting at toe and down sides. For
  center section shift of 2/3/2 changes direction of
  pattern.
Finish: Missing
Other: Structural padding on sole

192   Catalog no.: AR803 86.1
Site: Unknown
Collector and date: Probably Byron Cummings
  collection
Cultural period: Unknown
Construction technique: Plain weave
Dimensions: Length 18.5 cm, width 8.0 cm, depth
  1.0 cm
Active elements: Leaf element unspun, cortex intact
Average width: 0.53 cm
Passive elements: Leaf element unspun, cortex intact
Number of passive units: 2
Number in unit: 2
Average width: 0.81 cm
Ties, loops, attachments: Near instep two elements
  knot across sandal.
Shape: Rounded finished end
Start or Finish: Warps are tied together in two
  knots at toe.
Body: Over-under plain weave with narrow ends of
  leaf element on top and ending with shredded
  wide ends on sole for padding
Other: Structural padding on sole

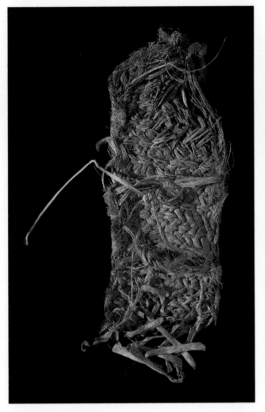

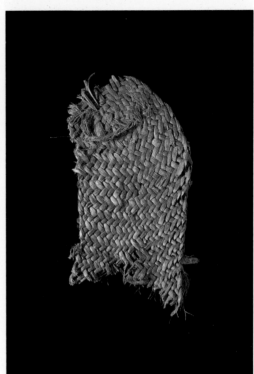

Catalog no.: AR939 86.1
Site: Unknown
Collector and date: Probably Byron Cummings
  collection
Cultural period: Unknown
Construction technique: Plaited
Dimensions: Length 29.5 cm, width 10.6 cm, depth
  1.20 cm
Active elements: Leaf elements unspun, cortex intact
Average width: 0.50 cm
Passive elements: N/A
Ties, loops, attachments: Toe: Two leaf elements
  intertwined and knotted. Edge: Remnants of ties
  and knots with one loop remaining on left side.
Shape: Right foot shaping, rounded toe, heel
  missing
Start: Active elements folded at toe
Body: 2/2 twill plaiting, drawing in near heel. At
  least 17 horizontal rows have been stitched on
  completed sandal. Stitches are long and short
  and appear only on upper surface indicating that
  the long stitches are back stitches and the short
  go only under surface wefts.
Finish: Heel missing but it appears elements
  remaining loop around adjacent elements.

Catalog no.: AR1847 87.1
Site: Unknown
Collector and date: Probably Byron Cummings
  collection
Cultural period: Unknown
Construction technique: Plaited
Dimensions: Length 17.65 cm, width 8.98 cm, depth
  0.85 cm
Active elements: Leaf element unspun, cortex intact
Average width: 0.40 cm
Passive elements: N/A
Ties, loops, attachments: Toe: Loop knotted on top
  of sandal, pierces sandal twice, loops over toe
  and pierces sandal twice again. Another loop of
  2 ply, s-Z twist cordage loops on sole of sandal
  with both ends protruding on upper side.
Shape: Right foot shaping, tapered toe, heel missing
Start: Active elements folded at toe with elements
  added as neccessary for tapering
Body: 2/2 twill plaiting for length of sandal. Element
  dropped near center for shaping. Exhausted ends
  left frayed on sole
Other: Structural padding on sole

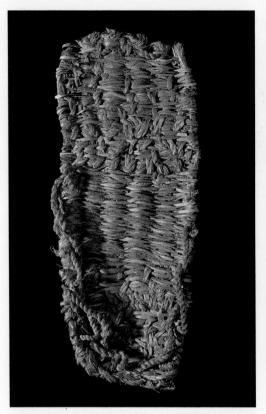

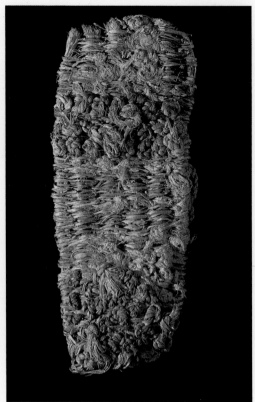

194   Catalog no.: AR1849 87.1
Site: Unknown
Collector and date: Probably Byron Cummings
    collection
Cultural period: Unknown
Construction technique: Plain weave
Dimensions: Length 18.5 cm, width 12.0 cm, depth
    .87 cm
Active elements: Leaf element unspun, partially
    decorticated
Average width: 0.34 cm
Passive elements: Shredded leaf elements 2 ply,
    lightly spun z and twisted together S
Number of passive units: 6
Number in unit: 1
Average width: 0.45 cm
Ties, loops, attachments: Toe: Remnants of cordage 2
    ply, s-Z twist. Heel and Edge: Cordage, 2 ply, s-Z
    twist, back stitched around heel and along both
    edges
Shape: Right foot shaping, squared toe, and cupped
    heel
Start: Warps are aligned parallel with ends
    extending beyond toe. Warps are anchored with
    one row of twining at toe.
Body: Over-under plain weave for length of sandal.
    At intervals of 12-14 rows a supplemental weft
    is woven for two rows. This is a leaf element,
    cortex intact.
Finish: At heel warp ends appear stitched back into
    body of sandal. Stitching at heel pulls in and
    forms a cupped heel.

Other: A pattern of knots for padding is made on
    the sole with a cordage 2 ply, s-Z twist with
    cortex partially intact. The cordage is stitched
    through sandal from the upper surface and
    knotted on the sole.

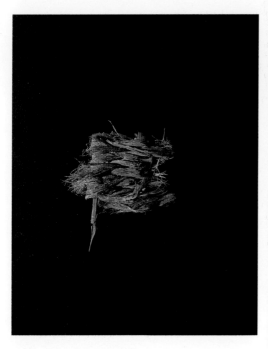

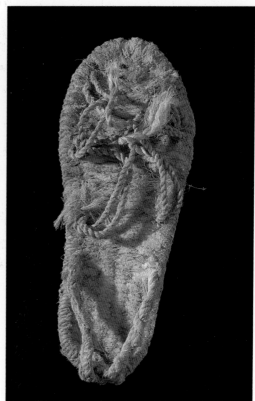

Catalog no.: AR1848 87.1
Site: Unknown
Collector and date: Probably Byron Cummings
collection
Cultural period: Unknown
Construction technique: Plain weave
Dimensions: Length 8.90 cm, width 6.60 cm, depth
1.6 cm
Active elements: Leaf element unspun, cortex intact
Average width: 0.42 cm
Passive elements: Leaf element unspun, cortex intact
Number of passive units: 2
Number in unit: 1
Average width: 0.42 cm
Ties, loops, attachments: None apparent
Shape: Unknown, fragmentary
Start or Finish: Missing
Body: Over-under plain weave with narrow ends of
leaf element on top and ending with shredded
wide ends on sole for padding
Other: Structural padding on sole. Charred

Catalog no.: AR 4006 94.1
Site: Unknown
Collector and date: Probably Byron Cummings
collection
Cultural period: Unknown
Construction technique: Plain weave
Dimensions: Length 27 cm, width 11 cm, depth 1.6
cm
Active elements: Shredded leaf element, twisted S
and Z
Average width: 0.45 cm
Passive elements: Cordage, 2 ply, s-Z twist
Number of passive units: 6
Number in unit: 1
Average width: 0.41 cm
Ties, loops, attachments: Edges: Two pieces of
cordage, 2 ply, s-Z twist, are used as one unit.
They loop and backstich along edges. Heel: Six
extended warps split into two to three warps
twist together on either side forming heel
attachment.
Shape: Right foot shaping, rounded toe, heel
cupped from warps pulled together
Start: Three cordage warps are folded at toe (one
inside the other) to form 6 warp elements.
Body: Tightly packed plain weave continues to heel.
Shredded yucca weft has been gathered together
for appropriate width of weft and twisted as it is
woven. This gives an "S" twist in one direction
and a "Z" in the opposite direction.
Finish: Two outer warps joined at heel in a knot.
Four inner warps divide and are each twisted
with one of the outer warps to form a heel
strap.

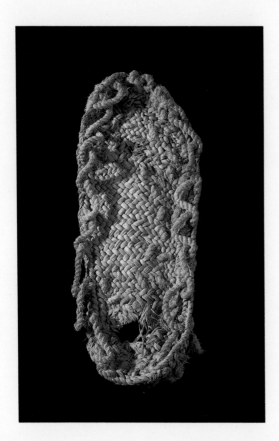

196   *Catalog no.:* AR4007 94.1
       Site: Unknown
       Collector and date: Probably Byron Cummings
          collection
       Cultural period: Unknown
       Construction technique: Plaited
       Dimensions: Length 24.5 cm, width 10.2 cm, depth
          0.58 cm
       Active elements: Leaf element unspun, cortex intact
       Average width: 0.38 cm
       Passive elements: N/A
       Ties, loops, attachments: Toe: Loops of cordage 2 ply,
          s-Z twist. Edges: Cordage 2 ply, s-Z twist, loops
          down both edges stitching into sandal 8-9 times.
       Shape: Right foot shaping, rounded toe and cupped
          heel
       Start: Active elements appear folded at toe
       Body: 2/2 twill plaiting, possible shifts. Cordage 2
          ply, s-Z twist stitched around heel, up right edge
          and across toe. Cordage twists on sole for each
          stitch, which creates a lug sole. Ends left frayed
          on sole
       Finish: Heel pulled in tightly for cupping. Active
          ends left protruding on sole
       Other: Structural padding on sole

BIBLIOGRAPHY

Adovasio, J. M., 1977. *Basketry Technology.* Chicago: Aldine Publishing.

Aikens, C. Melvin, 1986. "Jesse D. Jennings, Archaeologist." In *Anthropology of the Desert West: Essays in Honor of Jesse D. Jennings,* edited by Carol J. Condie and Don D. Fowler, pp. 3–5. University of Utah Anthropological Papers, no. 110. Salt Lake City: University of Utah Press.

Anderson, Keith M., 1969. "Tsegie Phase Technology." Ph.D. dissertation, Department of Anthropology, University of Washington, Seattle.

Ashley, Clifford W., 1949. *The Ashley Book of Knots.* Garden City, N.Y.: Doubleday.

Atkins, Victoria M., ed., 1993. *Anasazi Basketmaker.* Papers from the 1990 Wetherill–Grand Gulch Symposium. Cultural Resource Series no. 24. Salt Lake City: United States Department of the Interior, Bureau of Land Management.

Baldwin, Gordon C., 1938. "An Analysis of Basketmaker III Sandals from Northeastern Arizona." *American Anthropologist* 40:465–85.

Bell, Willis H., and Carl J. King, 1944. "Methods for the Identification of the Leaf Fibers of Mescal (*Agave*), Yucca (*Yucca*), Beargrass (*Nolina*), and Sotol (*Dasylirion*)." *American Antiquity* 1:150–60.

Byron Cummings Papers, 1860–1954, Trodden Trails, ACCN 1434, Manuscripts Division, Special Collections, University of Utah Marriott Library, Salt Lake City, Utah 84112.

Correll, Donovan Stewart, and Marshall Conring Johnston, 1979. *Manual of the Vascular Plants of Texas.* Richardson, Texas: University of Texas at Dallas.

Emery, Irene, 1966. *The Primary Structures of Fabrics.* Washington, D.C.: The Textile Museum.

Guernsey, Samuel James, 1931. *Explorations in Northeastern Arizona. Report on the Archaeological Fieldwork of 1920–1923.* Papers of the Peabody Museum of American Archaeology and Ethnology, vol. 12, no. 1. Cambridge, Mass.: Harvard University.

Guernsey, Samuel J., and A. V. Kidder, 1916. *Basket-Maker Caves of Northeastern Arizona. Report on the Explorations, 1916–1917.* Papers of the Peabody Museum of American Archaeology and Ethnology, vol. 8, no. 2. Cambridge, Mass.: Harvard University.

Gunnerson, James H., 1955. "Statewide Archaeological Survey." *Utah Archaeology* 1(1):3–4.

Harvey, Virginia I., 1978. *The Techniques of Basketry.* New York: Van Nostrand Reinhold.

Holloway, Richard G., 1991. *Identification of Cordage Remains from Site NA 5507, Antelope Cave, Arizona.* Castetter Laboratory for Ethnobotanical Studies, Technical Series Report no. 312. Provo, Utah: Museum of Peoples and Cultures, Brigham Young University.

Jennings, Jesse D., 1966. *Glen Canyon: A Summary.* University of Utah Anthropological Papers, no. 81. Salt Lake City: University of Utah Press.

———, 1969. *Operations Manual: Statewide Archaeological Survey.* Salt Lake City: University of Utah Archaeological Center.

Judd, Neil M., 1950. "Pioneering in Southwestern Archaeology." In *For the Dean: Essays in Anthropology in Honor of Byron Cummings,* edited by Erik K. Reed and Dale S. King, pp. 11–27. Hohokam Museum Association and Southwestern Monuments Association.

———, 1968. *Men Met Along the Trail: Adventures in Archaeology.* Norman: University of Oklahoma Press.

Kent, Kate Peck, 1957. *The Cultivation and Weaving of Cotton in the Prehistoric Southwestern United States.* Transactions of the American Philosophical Society, vol. 47, part 3. Philadelphia.

————, 1983. *Prehistoric Textiles of the Southwest.* Albuquerque: University of New Mexico Press.

Kidder, Alfred V., 1926. "A Sandal from Northeastern Arizona." *American Anthropologist* 28:618–32.

Kidder, Alfred V., and Samuel J. Guernsey, 1919. *Archeological Explorations in Northeastern Arizona.* Bureau of American Ethnology, Bulletin 65. Washington, D.C.: Smithsonian Institution.

Morris, Earl H., 1944. *Anasazi Sandals.* Clearing House for Southwestern Museums, *News-Letter* 68–69:239–41.

Morris, Elizabeth Ann, 1980. *Basketmaker Caves in Prayer Rock District, Northeastern Arizona.* Anthropological Papers no. 35. Tucson: University of Arizona Press.

Nusbaum, Jesse L., A. V. Kidder, and S. J. Guernsey, 1922. *A Basket Maker Cave in Kane County, Utah, with Notes on the Artifacts by A. V. Kidder and S. J. Guernsey.* Indian Notes and Monographs, Museum of the American Indian, Heye Foundation. New York.

Pepper, George H., 1902. *The Ancient Basket Makers of Southeastern Utah.* American Museum of Natural History, vol. 2, no. 4, Guide Leaflet no. 6. New York.

Robbins, Wilfred W., John P. Harrington, and Barbara Freire-Marreco, 1916. *Ethnobotany of the Tewa Indians.* Bureau of American Ethnology, Bulletin no. 55. Washington, D.C.

Rohn, Arthur H., 1971. *Mug House.* Archaeological Research Series no. 7-D, Washington, D.C.: National Park Service.

Smith, Elmer, 1955. "Utah Archaeology: An Outline of Its History." *Utah Archaeology* 1(2):2–7.

Stevenson, Matilda C., 1915. "Ethnobotany of the Zuni Indians." In *Thirtieth Annual Report of the Bureau of American Ethnology,* Washington, D.C.

Swank, George R., 1932. "The Ethnobotany of the Acoma and Laguna Indians." M.A. thesis, University of New Mexico, Albuquerque.

Tanner, Clara Lee, 1954. "Byron Cummings, 1860–1954." *The Kiva* 20(1):1–20.

————, 1976. *Prehistoric Southwestern Craft Arts.* Tucson: University of Arizona Press.

Webber, John Milton, 1953. *Yuccas of the Southwest.* Agriculture Monograph no. 17, U.S. Department of Agriculture, Washington, D.C.

CONTRIBUTORS

Artist *Margret Carde*, whose sketches of sandals, fragments, and interlacements grace this book, has an interest in prehistoric textiles that combines with her artistic talent to produce illustrations that entice the viewer to look closely at the inner workings of sandals.

Laurel Casjens, Curator of Collections at the Utah Museum of Natural History, is also a professional photographer whose talent is shown by the sandal photographs in this catalog.

Ann Hanniball is assistant director of the Utah Museum of Natural History.

Richard Holloway is professor of biology at the University of New Mexico. Among his many research projects are analyses of prehistoric plant, charcoal, fiber, and pollen remains.

Kathy Kankainen is Textile Laboratory supervisor and collections manager at the Utah Museum of Natural History.

Duncan Metcalfe, associate professor of anthropology at the University of Utah, is director of the University of Utah Archaeological Center and has been involved with many of the archaeological sites mentioned in this book.

Elizabeth Ann Morris, professor emerita at Colorado State University and daughter of the late Earl H. Morris, received her Ph.D. in anthropology from the University of Arizona. She has been deeply involved in the fields of archaeology and anthropology for many years. Her fieldwork and research include archaeological textiles and sandals.

Jay Nielsen of the Utah Museum of Natural History produced the detailed map of the Four Corners area where the sandals were collected.